POLIO

THOMAS ABRAHAM

Polio

The Odyssey of Eradication

HURST & COMPANY, LONDON

First published in the United Kingdom in 2018 by
C. Hurst & Co. (Publishers) Ltd.,
41 Great Russell Street, London, WC1B 3PL
© Thomas Abraham, 2018
All rights reserved.

Printed in India

The right of Thomas Abraham to be identified as the author
of this publication is asserted by him in accordance with the
Copyright, Designs and Patents Act, 1988.

Distributed in the United States, Canada and Latin America by
Oxford University Press, 198 Madison Avenue, New York, NY 10016,
United States of America.

A Cataloguing-in-Publication data record for this book
is available from the British Library.

ISBN: 9781849049566

This book is printed using paper from registered sustainable
and managed sources.

www.hurstpublishers.com

CONTENTS

CONTENTS

AUTHOR'S NOTE

Books about disease, and the efforts of men and women to protect human society from disease, tend to be written by epidemiologists, medical practitioners or historians of medicine. I belong to none of these professions.

Instead, this book is driven by an outsider's desire to understand one of the most ambitious acts that human society can undertake: to permanently rid the world of a disease by exterminating the pathogen that causes the disease. This technique, known as disease eradication, is controversial because it is prone to failure and it is expensive. But the potential benefits are great, and human beings are nothing if not optimistic. Which is why the campaign to stamp out polio began.

Disease is one of the many mirrors we can use to understand ourselves and the societies we live in. I have tried to use the trials and tribulations of the campaign to eradicate polio to look at some of the consequences of the unequal and divided world we live in.

In tracing the origins and the course of this campaign to eradicate polio, I have used the following sources: the rich lode of scientific papers that have been published on the virus; the vaccinatory and epidemiological course of the polio eradication campaign; the records of the World Health Organisation, particularly the debates and decisions of its Executive Board; the annual and semi-annual reports of the Global Polio Eradication Initiative (GPEI) and of its various advisory groups including the Independent Monitoring Board of the GPEI. I also consulted published histories of polio, and last but certainly not least, deployed the tools of my own profession of journalism. This involved visiting the frontlines of the polio campaign, as well as conducting interviews with key figures in the polio campaign.

This is not intended to be a comprehensive history of the polio campaign. That would require the work of a professional historian once the campaign is ended. Its aim is rather to cast an eye over the practice of global public health in a way that will hopefully provide food for thought when people embark upon future campaigns to control and eradicate disease on a global scale.

Thomas Abraham   April 2018

PROLOGUE

On a Saturday morning in early 2014 I found myself in the Karachi suburb of Gadap, a crowded labyrinth of brick and concrete tenements linked by narrow, dusty alleyways. A senior figure in the city administration, the Deputy District Commissioner, had come to inspect Karachi's troubled polio vaccination campaign and I had tagged along. With him was Dr Salah Tumseh, a voluble, energetic, Somali doctor who headed the World Health Organisation's (WHO's) polio campaign in the province. He in turn was followed by a train of lesser officials from the town health department, while an official photographer had come along to record the district administration at work.

Gadap is largely populated by migrants from the nearby provinces of Khyber Pakhtunkhwa and Balochistan. At the time I visited it was an epicentre of polio in Pakistan. Because it is migrants, rather than locals from the Sindh province, who live in these sprawling settlements on the margins of Karachi, the local government provides next to no services. If this is in the hope that the Pashtuns and Balochis will eventually go back to their home provinces, it hasn't worked. These people have lived here for generations in some cases, and all that official neglect has done is breed resentment. It's no coincidence that the Pakistan Taliban has been active in the area. We were close to where, in December 2012, the Taliban had shot dead four women polio vaccinators as they went to deliver drops to children. Two years on, the Taliban was still a threat, and our group was guarded by a phalanx of black clad paramilitary policemen cradling automatic weapons.

PROLOGUE

It was a Saturday morning, but there were few people around, and every door we passed was shut. The few residents we saw did not talk to or greet the officials, and none of the officials talked to them. Occasionally the procession stopped in front of a door and someone would knock to see if there were any children in the house and whether they had been vaccinated. Often, the doors would remain closed, but sometimes a door would open and a father would produce a child whose finger had been marked with ink by a polio vaccinator to show that the child had received polio drops. Parents had been threatened with arrest if they refused to allow their children to be immunised against polio, and the firmly shut doors reflected resentment.

A moment of reality pierced our passage through this sullen landscape when a door was flung open and a middle-aged man in a grimy singlet came out and wailed loudly to the passing river of officialdom. His wife was ill, he pleaded. Could someone please help him get her to a hospital? The Deputy District Commissioner stopped and listened gravely to the man's pleas, before informing him that they were there to inspect polio vaccination and could do nothing about his wife. Then he moved solemnly on with his retinue of officials and guards.

We made our way past closed doors until the roads petered out and we found ourselves on the banks of a fetid grey green canal. Gadap's sewage drained into it, and the thick sluggish mixture was almost certainly alive with poliovirus excreted by children. Given the prevalence of diarrhoeal diseases, the likelihood was also high that the canal was home to a flourishing community of viral and bacterial pathogens that could trickle into drinking water sources. This created a deadly chain of infection from water to sewage and back again.

The WHO representative, Dr Tumseh, gazed at the mess in front of him, and declared that he would try and get funding for water treatment machines to provide clean water. 'It is what people want and need', he said. Yet he knew that this was unlikely to happen on a scale large enough to make a difference. The polio campaign's focus was—and remains—to get polio drops into as many children as many times as possible. Tackling the wider environmental causes that allow polio and a host of other more serious diseases to flourish is beyond the polio campaign's mandate.

As I returned to central Karachi that afternoon, I was left with a sense of unease. The weapon-toting policemen, the closed doors, the

PROLOGUE

squalor, the sullen, unwelcoming population and the threat of violence
from the Taliban—these were not what I associated with a public health
campaign. Public health in modern times is regarded as a humanitarian,
egalitarian discipline, focused on responding to the health care needs of
communities. Marching with armed guards through deserted streets,
shut doors and unwelcoming householders did not appear to be the best
way to achieve public health targets. The polio campaign was doing its
best in extremely difficult circumstances to eradicate the poliovirus
through repeated vaccination campaigns. 'I have to chase the virus...
there is no way I can give [it] space to flourish,' declared Elias Durry, the
WHO's head of the polio programme in Pakistan at the time.

But forcing vaccines onto a resentful population—under threat from
the Taliban if they supported the polio programme and penalised by the
government if they did not get their children vaccinated—seemed to
go against the ethos of public health. It seemed an equally long way
from the cheerful posters of volunteers squeezing drops of vaccine into
the mouths of smiling children.

I also sensed in Karachi, and in other places in the world where polio
persisted, a bewilderment among the public at the attention given to
polio. To them it seemed a minor cause of illness among children compared to measles, malaria and diarrhoeal diseases. At the time I visited,
Pakistan was just recovering from a measles outbreak that had afflicted
several thousand children, and killed over 300. In contrast, there were
fifty-eight cases of polio, none of them fatal. Measles however did not
receive a fraction of the international attention that polio did.

Polio vaccinators would knock on people's doors week after week,
in repeated campaigns to give vaccines to the uncomprehending. Often
they were accompanied by armed policemen. In the case of other and
more serious illnesses, parents were left to their own devices. They
would have to spend money and get treated at private medical practitioners, or queue for long hours at underfunded government hospitals
and health centres.

It didn't help that the oral polio vaccine, the polio programme's tool
for eradication, was not as efficient in poor, densely populated parts of
the world as had been hoped. A schedule of two drops delivered twice
a year nationwide to children under the age of five was all that was
apparently needed to make the poliovirus disappear from a country.

But in practice, vaccine efficacy was extremely low in countries like India and Pakistan. So the WHO's strategy was to give doses of vaccine as many times as possible to children, regardless of how many times they had received drops earlier. In some states in India for example, children were being given ten to twelve doses of vaccine a year.

Parents were naturally puzzled, and later suspicious, about why governments, that otherwise provided little by way of health care, were so insistent that their children get repeated drops for a disease that, from their perspective, was rare. This suspicion in turn provided fertile ground for Islamic fundamentalist groups to argue that the vaccine was unsafe and was part of a Western plot against Muslims.

The fact is that polio eradication was a global imperative rather than a local one. Polio had been eliminated in most parts of the world, and so to keep these polio free areas safe, it was necessary that it be stamped out in pockets like Gadap, to remove the danger of the disease being re-imported. The people of Gadap were passive subjects in this larger global strategy. Their only role was to get their children immunised, or be threatened with arrest. Their children, their children's children and all future generations would of course benefit immensely by being protected from the crippling effects of polio. But it was hard for the public to see the benefit of this when more urgent health and developmental needs were not being met.

Ethically, the tactics that were being adopted in Pakistan to push polio vaccination would have been met with horror and public protest had they been used in wealthier parts of the world. If vaccinators in the United States, or Europe had knocked on peoples' doors and demanded that their children be immunised multiple times, this would have been seen as a serious breach of parental rights as well as of privacy. The threat of arrest if they did not vaccinate their children would have stoked outrage further. But because the people of Gadap were at the lowest end of the pecking order of global (even Pakistani) society, it was acceptable here.

The wheels of the polio programme were threatening to fall off. This was not just in the arid landscape of Karachi's bleak outlying suburbs, but—as I would discover—in other equally neglected parts of the world.

* * *

I first became aware of the global campaign to eradicate polio in 2009, the year I spent working at the WHO's headquarters in Geneva as a communications officer. In that same year an influenza pandemic swept the world and consumed much of the WHO's attention. Yet even amid the all-encompassing hubbub of the pandemic it was difficult to be unaware of the polio programme ticking away in the background, seemingly just a short step away from permanently wiping out the disease and liberating future generations. I was struck by the energy and determination of the polio team, as they ploughed relentlessly against the disease, berating governments in polio endemic countries to do a better job, and cajoling donors to keep funding the campaign.

I started to work on this book after I left the WHO. At first I thought the story would be an uncomplicated narrative of a battle against a disease. In the best epic tradition, it would have a cast of heroes (the polio fighters), villains (the virus and the people who rejected vaccination) and a climactic final battle in which the good guys win. The tale would be underpinned by a life-affirming message about the power of science and public health to help us lead healthier, happier lives.

But as I immersed myself in the details of the war on polio, the narrative morphed from a classic battle between heroes and villains to a more postmodern tale, shadowed in ambiguity and shrouded in multiple layers of meaning. Concepts that had appeared on first sight as clear and unambiguous as laws set in stone, on closer inspection became as slippery and elusive as a Zen koan. A simple history of the polio programme describing key figures and moments in the battle against the disease became a journey into a complex, multi-dimensional world where at times it seemed that nothing was quite as it seemed.

The public face of the polio programme is represented through cheerful posters of volunteers squeezing drops of oral polio vaccine into the mouths of children in Asia and Africa. Enthusiastic Rotarians generously donate their time as well as hundreds of millions of dollars to the cause, and celebrities endorse the programme. Yet the reality of the programme is best rendered in chiaroscuro. Shadows of failure mingle and give relief to bright areas of achievement.

As I unravelled the complexities of the polio programme—its failures, its achievements, its ethical ambiguities, its human heroism as well as its human failings—the story became even more admirable and fascinating. I began to discern the reality of what it meant to be in trench warfare against a resilient virus, using tools that were imperfect in conditions where there was often little or no support from governments or the public. Scientific and expert opinion was often divided. Powerful egos and interests would regularly collide, while geopolitical realities were as significant as science in determining success or failure.

The global polio eradication initiative is one of the most ambitious enterprises in the history of public health. Its aim is audacious: to exterminate the virus that causes polio, thereby permanently ridding the world of this disease. The virus in question is little more than a minute speck of genetic material, only perceivable under the most powerful of electron microscopes. Exterminating a virus requires that every single exemplar, in even the remotest corners in the world, must be tracked down, and stamped out. In the case of polio, the tool to achieve this is a vaccine that prevents the virus from infecting humans and replicating.

To attempt to control an infectious disease by exterminating its cause is known as eradication. It is the most difficult way to protect humans against a disease but the most permanent. The technical challenges posed by disease eradication make it medical science's equivalent of landing a man on the moon. The risks of failure are high: the world has embarked on six disease eradication campaigns over the last 100 years. Of them, only one, smallpox has succeeded. Expensive, decade-long campaigns against malaria and yellow fever ended in failure, while the fate of the polio campaign, though close to success, remains up in the air. Yet it is a tribute to human optimism that disease eradication is still seen as a viable strategy. If polio is eradicated, there is little doubt that measles will be the next target.

In May 1988, when the WHO's member countries passed a resolution calling for polio to be eradicated by the year 2000 as 'a gift from the twentieth to the twenty-first century', the consensus was that this was an achievable target. A cheap, effective, easy to use oral vaccine existed, and a recently launched regional campaign in the countries of South America had shown rapid and remarkable success. All that needed to be done was to take this experience and expand it to the rest of the world.

Initially, the optimism appeared well-founded. Across the world, in fits and starts, countries launched twice yearly national immunisation days, during which children would be fed polio vaccine. The campaigns were not always well organised, and often numbers of children were missed. But such was the power of the vaccine, that even these often poorly conducted vaccination campaigns were enough to stamp out the virus across large parts of the globe.

In 1988, before the eradication campaign was launched, the WHO estimated there were around 350,000 new cases of polio every year, spread over 125 countries. By 2000, there were only an estimated 2,880 cases a year, spread over twenty countries. While the year 2000 deadline to eradicate polio had been missed, the numbers of new cases, as well as the geographic extent of the virus had shrunk like a tumour retreating in the face of a miracle cancer drug. And if we look behind these abstract figures, we see hundreds of thousands of healthy, physically able children who might otherwise have caught polio but for these efforts.

This alone would count for a major victory in the annals of public health. If, even despite these achievements, the polio programme is still haunted by the possibility of failure it is because of the very scale of its ambition: to eradicate, or wipe from the earth the virus that causes the disease.

Success in an eradication campaign is measured not by a dramatic reduction of the disease to a minor public health problem in a few pockets of the world, but by the complete extinction of the pathogen causing the disease. As Fred Soper, a key figure in the eradication campaigns against malaria and yellow fever in the early twentieth century put it, 'eradication is an absolute'.[1]

Disease eradication is a powerful and compelling idea. With successful eradication, there is one less disease for future generations to worry about. The idea of never having to worry about smallpox, or ever having to see a child crippled by polio goes to the heart of what public health should be. In addition, the economic benefits of eradicating a widely prevalent disease are potentially enormous as routine vaccination against the disease will no longer be necessary. In the case of the polio programme, the benefits to the world once the disease is eradicated and vaccination can be stopped, is estimated to be around US$1.5 billion a year.

However, disease eradication remains a contentious idea in the world of public health. The costs are high as are the risks of failure. And it is not as though eradication is the only way to protect people from disease. Many diseases that were major causes of sickness and death just 100 years ago, such as diphtheria and measles, have virtually disappeared in the modern world because of vaccination (though measles has made a comeback in the West because of the anti-vaccine movement). These diseases are not threats anymore, even though the pathogens that cause them still exist in nature.

Eradication may be the permanent solution to a disease, but many would argue that given the expense of an eradication campaign, and the uncertainty over success, disease control programmes are the more practical solution to reducing cases of polio globally.

One of the arguments in favour of eradicating polio, is that it is only one of a handful of diseases that can be eradicated. Diseases caused by pathogens that exist only in humans can be eradicated, provided a good vaccine to immunise against the disease exists. Polio meets both essential criteria: the poliovirus can only replicate in humans, and there are vaccines effective enough to make sure that the virus can no longer replicate. This provides a strong chance of the eventual extinction of the virus.

Proponents of eradication take the view that if a disease meets the criteria for eradication, then global health organisations have an ethical and moral obligation to do so. As the late Ciro de Quadros, the Brazilian epidemiologist who was one of the guiding spirits of the polio eradication campaign put it to me, 'If you can eradicate, you should eradicate. No ifs and buts…'

But others such as the late Carl Taylor, a professor of public health at Johns Hopkins University and an expert on health systems in developing countries, had a different take. Taylor believed that while polio eradication would bring immense benefits to future generations, focusing on this single disease needed to be balanced against many more common threats to health and life. 'Poor countries naturally give priority to problems such as pneumonia, malaria, diarrhoea, measles and malnutrition,' he said. Taylor went on to ask a question that I found highly pertinent after my travels through the countries where polio persisted. 'Should poor countries, with many health problems that could be controlled, divert their limited resources for a global goal that has low priority for their own children?'[2]

Other prominent figures in international public health concur. In a 2012 essay, experts including Julio Frenk, dean of the Harvard School of Public Health and Peter Piot, former head of the UN Aids programme, wrote that single disease eradication programmes were unhelpful when people faced multiple health issues. 'The focus on specific diseases has imposed and exposed fault lines in delivering services in places where many suffer from multiple health issues at the same time or at varying points in their lives,' they declared.[3] Like others in the world of public health, they argued for a more integrated approach focused on the health of a person or community, rather than a silo-based approach focused on a specific disease. What I saw in Pakistan, and elsewhere on the polio trail seemed to support this view. Clean water, sanitation, protection against measles, malaria and diarrhoea were more important to the public than polio was, and an integrated approach might have won greater public acceptance.

In fact, the original decision by the World Health Assembly in 1988, made it clear that polio eradication was to be part of a larger WHO programme known as the Expanded Programme of Immunisation (EPI), to vaccinate the world's children against a number of common diseases. Polio eradication was not to be an end in itself, but an approach to the broader goal of reaching children with a variety of vaccines against childhood diseases. Eradication efforts 'should be pursued in ways that strengthen the EPI as a whole, fostering its contribution, in turn, to the development of the health infrastructure and of primary health care,' the resolution declared.

Behind the tangled prose lay a powerful idea. Instead of running a traditional eradication campaign that attacked a single disease, why not use the polio campaign to strengthen other healthcare services as well as delivering further childhood vaccines? This would ensure that children were better protected not merely against polio, but against all the key diseases that threatened them.

The polio programme however quickly broke out of what it perceived as the straitjacket imposed on it by having to work alongside other vaccination programmes. It began to follow its own path as a largely autonomous campaign, focused solely on distributing polio vaccine through door-to-door campaigns. This initially happened because of increasing impatience within the polio programme and among donors at the slow pace at which eradication was proceeding. Part of the reason for the slowness, the polio programme felt, was that it was being boxed in and losing focus by being tied down by other immunisation campaigns. The only way to forge ahead and complete the job of immunisation was to break free.

Initially, this strategy of going it alone worked well. The polio eradication campaign, as we have seen, succeeded in eliminating polio from large parts of the world through intense twice-yearly (or often more frequent) vaccination drives during which every child in the country was given polio drops. But the weakness of going it alone became apparent when time and time again countries where polio had disappeared were re-infected. This was because the polio campaign had not worked alongside health departments in these countries to strengthen routine childhood vaccination. This meant that infants would not receive regular polio vaccine after the country-wide vaccination drives had ended.

On top of this, while fresh outbreaks of polio recurred at regular intervals in polio-free countries, proving a great cause for worry in the eradication campaign, there was a still greater cause for concern. From time to time these outbreaks were being caused by the polio vaccine itself.

* * *

If vaccines could talk, the oral polio vaccine could well reveal itself as a god from Greek mythology: blessed with miraculous powers, but also possessed of a fatal weakness. The oral vaccine that Albert Sabin, developed in the late 1950s had near miraculous power in clearing wide parts of the world of the poliovirus in a relatively short time. Yet the vaccine was based on a live, but weakened poliovirus. On rare occasions it could cause polio which spread through communities in exactly the same way that natural, or wild, polioviruses did.

The WHO and the polio campaign had been aware of this problem since 2000, when a vaccine-derived polio outbreak was identified on the island of Hispaniola in the Caribbean. In the years that followed, several polio cases caused by the vaccine were detected in other places in the world. The most devastating was in Nigeria, where over 400 children were paralysed by multiple instances of polio caused by the vaccine virus between 2005 and 2011. Between 2000 and mid-2017, the polio eradication campaign recorded over 831 cases of children who had been paralysed in outbreaks of vaccine derived polio occurring in twenty-seven countries. This was not something that the polio campaign publicised. To do so would have destroyed public confidence in the campaign, donor money would have dried up, and the eradication would have failed. The WHO also felt it had no alternative to using the oral polio vaccine if eradication was to be achieved.

Another vaccine did exist: an injected killed virus vaccine of the kind first developed by American virologist Jonas Salk, which was far safer than the oral polio vaccine. But it was also more expensive, and there were fears that the campaign would not be able to raise enough money to meet vaccine costs. It also needed trained health workers to inject children, which meant that poor countries might find it difficult to run vaccination campaigns. Perhaps most importantly, while the injected vaccine protected a child from getting polio, it did not prevent a child from transmitting polio to others, which made it an imperfect tool for eradication. These arguments against the injected vaccine would be contested by outside experts, but the dominant WHO view prevailed.

The outbreaks of polio caused by the vaccine were rationalised as collateral damage. Just as unintended casualties occur in a war when an enemy is attacked, so were children occasionally paralysed by the vaccine. Yet it was argued that these cases of paralysis, numbering in the hundreds, needed to be balanced against the millions of children whom the vaccine was protecting against paralysis.

The Sabin vaccine in fact caused paralysis in two distinct ways. One way, as described above, was when the normally benign, weakened polio virus that the vaccine contained started spreading in communities with low immunisation rates and reacquired mutations that caused paralysis. This was known as polio caused by a circulating vaccine-derived polio virus (cVDPV), and was first observed in 2000. Another route by which the Sabin vaccine caused paralysis had been known since the time the vaccine went into use in North America in the 1960s. In one in every million or so children who received the vaccine, because of as yet unknown factors, the vaccine virus paralysed the child (or in some cases parents or siblings to whom the child transmitted the vaccine virus). This was known as vaccine associated paralytic polio

(VAPP). In all of these cases, the paralysis caused by the vaccine was indistinguishable from that caused by the natural poliovirus. This weakness in the oral polio vaccine has been extensively documented in the scientific literature and the WHO estimated that between 250–500 children a year had contracted VAPP and been paralysed by the oral polio vaccine.[4]

But to the world at large, including parents in India, Pakistan, Nigeria and other parts of the developing world, the oral vaccine was portrayed as a safe, effective way to prevent polio.

When I first began work on this book, there was nothing in any of the material that the polio campaign put out for the public, or anything that campaign spokespeople said that indicated that the vaccine could cause a problem. There was a wealth of scientific studies in technical journals, and the issue was discussed at length in internal meetings. But none of this trickled down to the public, except through occasional acknowledgments that in rare instances the polio vaccine could cause paralysis.

Within the polio eradication campaign itself, there was a feeling that the problems caused by outbreaks of vaccine-derived virus were secondary to the main goal of eradicating wild poliovirus. The oral polio vaccine was the most effective way of stopping transmission, and had to be continued. It was argued that once the natural poliovirus was stamped out, the problem of vaccine-derived polioviruses could be looked at, provided they still continued to occur. But to those outside the world of public health, the idea that a vaccine that could cause the disease it was meant to protect against was difficult to come to terms with.

The problems caused by vaccine-derived polioviruses are a perfect example of the messy reality that lies underneath an ambitious global health campaign, a reality the public rarely sees. The public face of the polio campaign is one of unvarying optimism, and the public narrative goes as follows: the oral polio vaccine is safe, effective, easy to administer and the perfect tool for eradication. Through the heroic efforts of volunteers and polio workers, children in even the most inaccessible places of the world are being reached. It's only a matter of time before the campaign succeeds. Bruce Aylward, for more than a decade the head of the polio programme in the WHO, and an articulate spokesperson for the campaign, gave a perfect example of the campaign's can-do spirit at a

TED talk in 2011. 'With a combination of smart technologies and smart investments, polio can now be eradicated anywhere...we have the chance to write an entirely new polio-free chapter in human history.'[5]

At the time of writing—eight years after that TED talk—the poliovirus still persists in Pakistan, Afghanistan and perhaps Nigeria. In addition, outbreaks of vaccine-derived poliovirus are regularly cropping up in countries that were believed to have been polio-free. One of the most urgent challenges facing the polio campaign now is to end the use of oral polio vaccine. It needs to be replaced with an inactivated, killed virus polio vaccine that will protect against vaccine-derived polioviruses that might still cause polio even though the natural poliovirus has been eradicated.

* * *

Eckard Wimmer has spent the best part of a scientific career that spans over half a century studying and probing the mysterious existence of viruses. A German-born biochemist, who has lived in the United States since the 1960s, Wimmer is a genial, courteous man. He likes to tease visitors to his laboratory at Stonybrook University on Long Island with a question: is a virus living or non-living? As I helplessly ponder this, Wimmer comes to my rescue, explaining the paradox that has fascinated him for most of his professional life. Viruses occupy a twilight zone between chemistry and biology: at times they are living, replicating particles, and at other times, they are inert chemicals. Until they infect a living host, they are nothing but chemicals, incapable of reproduction, and lacking in any of the characteristics that biologists would use to define life. But once they infect a living cell, they come to life in the cell, taking over its machinery and turning it into a factory to reproduce billions of new viral particles.

Wimmer is a distinguished polio virologist, and I have come to see him to try to understand the implications of an experiment that has brought him some notoriety in the scientific community. In 2002, Wimmer and his associates at Stonybrook took the idea that a virus outside a host is nothing more than a complex chemical molecule (in the case of the poliovirus $C_{332,652} H_{492,388} N_{98,245} O_{131,196} P_{7,501} S_{2340}$) to its logical conclusion. They synthesised a poliovirus in the laboratory using commercially available sequences of DNA. The team then created a

DNA copy of the virus genome (the poliovirus is an RNA virus), converted that into an RNA version using easily available enzymes, placed the enzymes in a growth medium and watched as the RNA particles assembled and replicated to become infectious poliovirus particles.

Wimmer had created a lethal virus in his laboratory using commonly obtainable material, and methods that anyone with basic laboratory skills could follow. Not surprisingly there was outrage and concern among the scientific community and the public, at a time when fears of bioterrorism were widespread following the 9/11 attacks. One biologist described it in a letter to *Science* magazine as a 'stunt' and worried that it would merely heighten public fears about bioterrorism, and fears that deadly pathogens would be synthesised in laboratories and released into the world.[6]

In fact Wimmer's motives were more scientific. He wished to demonstrate that viruses could be regarded as chemicals, and so could be synthesised in labs with commercially available materials. As he noted in response to the criticisms, by 2005, technologies in synthetic biology had progressed to such an extent that it would be possible, at least theoretically to synthesise the poliovirus at the cost of a few cents, and more complex viruses like ebola for a few dollars in the laboratory. It was important for people to take note of this.

Wimmer's work is relevant to the polio eradication project because if the poliovirus (and other pathogens) can be synthesised in a laboratory, then eradication, as a permanent solution, suddenly seems a little less permanent. He has warned that it would be dangerous to ever stop immunising children against polio, because it could always be artificially created and released back into society by anyone with undergraduate level laboratory skills and malign intent. 'The new reality of rapid *de novo* synthesis of viruses forces us to ask whether the polio campaign has been rendered a dream,' he wrote.

The polio programme did not take this prospect very seriously, but if viruses can be synthesised in laboratories, it does raise the question of whether true eradication is ever possible. Will it ever be wise to stop vaccinating children against a disease even after the pathogen that causes it has disappeared from nature?

* * *

PROLOGUE

As I travelled through the last battlefields of the war against polio in northern Nigeria and Pakistan, talking to government officials, it was apparent that these countries would have paid no attention to polio eradication without international pressure. Polio was not a priority for their governments or for the public. It was the WHO, UNICEF, the Gates Foundation, the US Centers for Disease Control and Prevention (CDC) and Rotary International—the organisations leading the global polio eradication campaign—that were pushing these countries to act.

Often these international organisations felt they were hitting their heads against a brick wall. At every level of government, whether it was at the national, state, district or village level, officials were unconvinced of the need to give polio priority over other diseases. At the lower levels of government, district and village officials were happy to take the funding that polio brought (and there was no shortage of credible accounts of polio money being pocketed by officials in both countries). But they saw little need to act with the urgency or efficiency that the polio campaign needed to succeed.

At the highest levels of government though, officials and ministers were much more amenable to international pressure, since their country's reputations were at stake. At international meetings, heads of state would be regularly chided for their failure to contain polio, and reminded to do their duty. One such occasion was on 27 September 2012, during the United Nations General Assembly in New York when the then UN Secretary-General, Ban Ki Moon, hosted a lunchtime gathering. He had brought together Aseef Zardari, Hamid Karzai, and Goodluck Jonathan, the leaders of Pakistan, Afghanistan and Nigeria—three remaining countries where polio was still prevalent. Bill Gates, one of the principal funders of the polio eradication campaign, was also in attendance, along with the heads of the WHO and UNICEF, Rotary International, and other representatives from donor governments.

The meeting aimed to drum up financial support for the polio programme, keep flagging spirits alive, ensure polio was still in the public eye, and maintain the pressure on the three presidents to complete eradication. The mood was set by a short film at the opening. This interspersed shots of the moon landing, Nelson Mandela's release from prison in South Africa, and the fall of the Berlin Wall, leaving no doubts about the scale of historic endeavour that eradicating polio was deemed to be.

PROLOGUE

The three presidents, each battling civil unrest along with a host of social and economic problems, assured the gathering they were fully committed to polio eradication. All made the right noises, ('Afghanistan will try hard and hard and surely we will win,' declared Karzai). But there was also a sense that they had been hauled before a tribunal of the rich and powerful and told to get a job done, because the world needed them to do it. The presidents read out from a list of measures they had taken, detailed the problems they faced and repeatedly asserted they would get the job done. It was telling that Karzai also revealed that he had not even been aware there would be this meeting at the UN on polio until Bill Gates had phoned him in Kabul to talk about the polio programme.

The speeches and declarations from the donors and the organisations running the programme were upbeat and exhortatory. Eradicating polio was a mission that had to succeed in order to remove this blight from the lives of children forever. All that was needed was for the countries involved to make that extra little effort to wipe the poliovirus from the remaining districts in which it existed, by reaching children who had not been vaccinated so far.

'Failure to eradicate polio is unforgiveable...failure is not an option,' declared the WHO's then Director-General, Margaret Chan. The moral and ethical imperative to eradicate a disease that was so close to extinction was a common theme in the speeches. 'This is a noble cause,' Gates said, adding that funding the polio programme was the smartest use of resources that the world could make. Anthony Lake, the head of UNICEF, said it would be hard to think of a greater injustice than to allow the poliovirus to continue to cripple children in the future.

Such commitment and clarity of purpose is admirable, as is the self-belief and determination to succeed. Everyone involved is given the sense of being part of an important global crusade. Questions about how relevant this emphasis on eradicating a single disease is for these three countries—and whether it would not make more sense to combine this effort with other public health programmes—are made to seem petty and carping. It does not seem to matter that polio is not a major disease threat in these countries. Nor is it taken into account that if the people the programme is targeting had any say in the matter, they would probably have asked for the money to be spent on more urgent health needs.

The challenges of ensuring that vaccine-derived viruses do not lead to fresh outbreaks are not mentioned. The emphasis is on pushing ahead and getting the job done. Perhaps this determination to succeed no matter what is an essential ingredient for any endeavour this large and ambitious.

But for the detached observer, Gadap in Pakistan and the United Nations headquarters in New York may as well be on different planets. The declarations made by the leaders of the polio eradication programme seem to have little resonance with the reality of the lives lived by villagers in Nigeria, Pakistan and Afghanistan, or millions of other places in the developed world. Their voices are unheard in New York and other places where the powerful congregate to deliberate and decide the fate of the world.

On a visit to Nigeria in 2012, in a small village called Marke in Kano province, I heard a local farmer called Sabiu angrily ask a polio vaccination team what seemed to be a universal question. 'Why do you keep coming again and again to give polio vaccine? Why this polio, polio?'

This book is an attempt to answer this question on behalf of Sabiu and countless others. Why polio, polio? How did this disease, a relatively minor cause of illness and death among children become the focus of a major global health programme and receive so much more attention than other diseases?

The answer lies partly in how the disease was experienced in the most powerful country in the world, the United States in the last century. This had a strong impact on globally framing polio as a disease that was particularly dreadful, and could and should be stamped out. Franklin Delano Roosevelt, president of the United States during the momentous period of the depression of the 1930s and the war years of the 1940s, was a polio survivor. He put his considerable political clout into helping frame polio as a disease that could be defeated, and into raising funds for polio that would lead to the creation of two vaccines.

Yet the real battle against polio globally was not in the United States or Europe, but in the developing world, where poverty, poor health services, poor sanitation and often violent social conflicts created conditions in which the poliovirus thrived. These were also parts of the world that did not share the terrible memories of polio epidemics that the developed world did: polio was just another disease, and giving it priority over other diseases made little sense to people. Increasingly the battle against polio was seen as a Western-inspired battle, carried out by international organisations and groups that were funded by the world's rich countries as well as one of the world's richest men, Bill Gates. I focus on the problems the polio eradication campaign faced in Pakistan and India to illustrate this clash between health programmes decided and conceived in the world's centres of power, and the needs and aspirations of those in developing countries.

This is also the story of the battle between a virus and a vaccine. It is about man's efforts to exterminate the poliovirus using a vaccine that is based on a weakened form of the poliovirus. The Sabin vaccine is a remarkable creation designed to mimic the wild poliovirus and push it out of the only environment it can reproduce in: the human intestines. But polioviruses have evolved over millennia to survive, and will exploit any weakness or gap to survive. So, as the polio hunters have chased the virus across the globe, swatting away at it with vaccine, the virus has found new niches in which to survive, niches caused by poverty, conflict and human misery. To complicate matters, the vaccine virus has the same biological imperative to survive as its natural cousin, and has gone off in surprising directions of its own.

The narrative of polio eradication presented by the WHO and its partners, UNICEF and Rotary, is always straightforward and cheerfully optimistic. The polio campaign is doing the right thing, the vaccine works excellently, and we are just a heartbeat away from wiping out a disease forever. But eradication—which was due to have been completed in 2000—is already eighteen years over schedule, and each additional year has cost approximately US$1 billion that could have been spent on other urgent health issues. Eradicating polio has proved to be a long, hard, costly battle and this book is an attempt to understand why.

The campaign to eradicate polio was launched in 1988. But this would not have been possible without decades' work from scientists to understand the virus that caused the disease, how the virus spread between humans and the way it affected the nerves of the spinal cord to cause paralysis. It would not have been possible without a huge national effort in the most powerful country in the world in the twentieth century, the United States, to fund scientific knowledge of polio and polio vaccines. This national effort was, understandably, sparked primarily by the experience of polio in the United States. Yet to fully understand the drive to conquer polio, we need first to understand the precise nature of the disease, the virus that causes it, and the vaccines that were created to conquer the virus.

PART I

THE VIRUS, THE VACCINE
AND A CRIPPLED PRESIDENT

1

THE SHADOWY WORLD OF THE POLIOVIRUS

For more than two decades, Dr Mathew Varghese has performed reconstructive surgery on the twisted limbs of polio patients, and so has deeper knowledge than most of the cruel impact that the poliovirus can have on people's bodies and lives. As I sit with him in his cramped office at St Stephen's Hospital in Delhi, Varghese flips through before and after photographs of patients on his laptop. A typical image shows a young woman after almost a year of surgery and recovery, standing and smiling at the camera, her weakened limbs supported by braces hidden under her clothing.

'She came to me when she was 18, and she was carried in by her father on his back... almost like a backpack. Both her legs were paralysed and deformed, and she had never walked in her life. I operated on both her knees, both her hips, both her ankles.' The procedures were long, and the recovery was painful. But it allowed the young woman to regain what Varghese sees an essential element of being human: the ability to stand upright on her own two feet.

Varghese runs what is probably one of the last hospital wards in India dedicated to reconstructive surgery for polio. Polio has disappeared from the country, and his remaining patients are not young children, but young adults, in their late teens and early twenties, who were crippled as infants, but have only now come for surgery. 'It is when they start thinking of getting married that they come here,' he says.

The poliovirus does not directly affect the limbs. It infects and kills cells in the anterior horn of the spinal column, a part of the spine that contains the motor neurons that control the muscles of our limbs. When these cells die, the muscles of the limbs they control atrophy, and as the limbs fall into disuse, they shrink and become deformed and twisted.

Some patients come to Varghese able only to crawl. Others can stand upright with crutches. Others can hobble along with callipers. 'I try to get them up the step ladder of mobility. If someone comes who can only crawl, I try and get them upright. If someone comes to me able to walk with crutches, I try and get them off the crutches. If someone comes with a calliper or brace, I see if I can eliminate the brace. If a patient can walk without a brace but has a limp, I see if I can make the limp better.'

As Varghese describes his surgical procedures, the images that come to my mind are of an engineering workshop. Twisted bones are surgically broken and then straightened and stretched over months in a technique known as distraction. When a leg is too short, the bones are cut and then lengthened by several centimetres using an external fixation device known as the Ilizarov apparatus. In other cases deformed limbs are straightened with plaster casts and screws that are gradually tightened till they are straight enough.

Varghese, an ascetic looking man with a startling resemblance to photographs of Gandhi in his younger days, is one of a dying breed of physicians and surgeons for whom medicine is a moral calling rather than a road to riches. There is little doubt in his mind that polio needs to be eradicated, despite the multiple other health challenges that poor societies face. 'This disease is preventable, this deformity is preventable, the disability is preventable, yet as a society, we just have not done enough,' he says.

Varghese finds polio a particularly distressing disease, because it strikes at two essential elements that define what it means to be a human. Polio affects the nerves that control the quadriceps, the muscle in the front of our thighs that make it possible for humans to walk upright. It also affects the muscles that make fine motor control possible, two skills that divide homo sapiens from nearly all other forms of life. 'In the evolution of mankind, the last muscle that evolved was the quadriceps, that allowed man to stand upright. This was the last muscle in our evolution, and polio affects the last muscle in our evolution.' Similarly, when polio affects the hands and arms, the two muscles that are commonly paralysed are the muscle that allows us to raise our arms, and the muscle that allows us to pinch and make fine movements with our fingers. 'The ability to make fine movements is essential to homo sapiens', he says.

As he walks me out of the hospital, he ruminates on the theme of the poliovirus' ability to destroy its victim's humanity, and the physical as well as mental toll this can take. 'Imagine the stigma it causes, the stigma of deformity, the stigma of crutches.' As I depart, he advises me to read the work of the Canadian-American sociologist Erving Goffman on stigma to understand the full extent of the social disability that a polio patient faces.

* * *

Polio is thought to be an ancient disease, and the poliovirus is believed to be among the oldest viruses that have afflicted humans, though evidence of its antiquity is of necessity patchy and inconclusive. A carving from the Egyptian eighteenth dynasty (1403–1365 BC), now in the Ny Carlsberg Glyptotek in Copenhagen, shows a young man with a withered and shortened right leg holding a long stick for support, the right foot drooping in a manner suggestive of poliomyelitis. The Greek physician, Hippocrates, writing around 1,000 years later in his characteristic style that blended descriptions of the environment and climate with disease, described an outbreak of paralytic sickness on the island of Thasos. 'The summer was hot,' he wrote. 'This hot spell began suddenly, and was both continuous and severe. There was no rain... about the time of Arcturus southerly rains began and continued till the equinox... under such circumstances, cases of paralysis started to appear during the winter and became common, constituting an epidemic. Some cases were swiftly fatal.'[1] Other evidence, from Egyptian mummies to descriptions of the Roman Emperor Claudius' maladies, has been cited as evidence of ancient poliomyelitis infections.[2]

Though the poliovirus appears to have infected humans from the earliest times, for many centuries it did not seem to have caused epidemics. Michael Underwood, an English paediatrician writing in 1789, described polio as being not uncommon among children, but did not report epidemics sweeping through the population. It was only in the nineteenth century in Europe, and then in the early twentieth century in the United States that polio was transformed from a disease that affected individual children to one that reached epidemic scale. One of the earliest outbreaks of the disease was recorded in 1881 in Sweden by a doctor in Västerbotten province, who reported clusters of children and teenagers being struck by a paralytic disease he described as polio-myelitis anterior acuta.[3] By the early twentieth century, epidemics of the disease had become regular features of the summer in Sweden and other parts of Scandinavia, and had soon spread across the Atlantic to the United States. Summer epidemics of polio terrified parents and children, especially at a time when better hygiene and sanitation had sharply reduced the toll of many other infectious diseases.

Finding the cause of this disease and understanding how it spread became a major focus of medical science. Not surprisingly, early attempts to identify the cause of polio were marked by several excursions into blind alleys. At first it was not even clear that a microbe caused polio. Swedish parents used to advise children not to kick the leaves that fell on the ground during the late summer and early autumn months, or even eat apples that fell on the ground. They believed that it was some sort of miasma, or bad air collecting in leaves that caused the disease.[4]

Part of the mystery was that there were often no visible chains of transmission from one patient to another. Some children would get paralysed, while friends and family members with whom they were in close contact would remain disease-free, an unusual pattern for an infectious disease that seemed to travel rapidly through communities.

Meticulous work by the Swedish physician Ivar Wickman in 1907 solved the riddle of why there were often no clear chains of transmission. Many, perhaps most children infected with polio showed no signs of disease, but could pass the virus onto others who would develop paralysis.

If the disease was infectious (and not everyone was convinced of this at the time) the consensus appeared to be that it was bacterial rather than viral. Many scientists saw parallels between polio and epidemics of meningitis. In 1887 the Viennese bacteriologist Anton Weichselbaum isolated the bacteria that caused meningococcal disease, and sparked a futile hunt to identify a similar bacterium in the fluids and tissues of polio patients. Injecting blood and tissue from polio patients into the usual laboratory animals—rabbits, guinea pigs and mice—failed to produce disease in these creatures. As the Yale University physician John Paul wrote in his magisterial history of polio, 'for nearly a generation a fruitless search had been going on to find such a microbial agent (for polio). Numerous false hopes had been raised by claimants who championed this or that species of bacteria.'[5]

It fell to another Viennese scientist, Karl Landsteiner, a former assistant to Weicheslbaum, to demonstrate polio's viral origins, and as in many scientific breakthroughs luck appeared to play a part. In November 1908, a nine-year-old Viennese boy died of polio and Landsteiner and his assistant Erwin Popper ground up samples from the boy's spinal cord. They then filtered it to remove any bacteria, and injected the fluid into laboratory mice, rabbits and guinea pigs, but with no effect. Unusually, Landsteiner had access to two monkeys that had been acquired for experiments on syphilis. Monkeys were expensive and would not normally have been available for rather routine attempts to identify the cause of polio. The two monkeys were of different species, but both reacted after being injected with the ground spinal cord. One of them died eight days after the injection, but showed no observable signs of paralysis before it died. The other monkey developed polio-like paralysis in both its legs after seventeen days.

In December 1908 at a Medical Congress in Vienna, Landsteiner and Erwin displayed slides from the spinal cords of the two monkeys and the one human case. All three of them displayed identical lesions, convincing the audience that it was indeed polio that had killed the monkeys, and that the infectious agent had been present in spinal cord suspension drawn from the human victim. Given that the suspension was free of bacteria, the obvious conclusion, given the lack of any other techniques at the time to either see or cultivate viruses, was that polio was viral in origin. Later, Landsteiner used spinal cord material from the two infected monkeys to pass the infection to other monkeys, all of which developed characteristic polio lesions in their spinal cords—further proof that polio was caused by an infectious agent.

Polio was becoming an increasingly significant public health threat in Europe and the United States, and Landsteiner's discovery opened the gates to a wave of new research into the disease and its methods of transmission. He went on to collaborate with Constantin Levaditi, a Romanian physician and microbiologist at the Pasteur Institute, to try and understand how the poliovirus got into the nervous system. They began searching for traces of the virus in other human tissues to see if they could find a pathway of entry to the spinal cord. They tested tissue from non-fatal polio cases and found traces of the virus in the throat, salivary glands and in the intestinal lymph nodes. This was an important clue to the way the poliovirus entered its human host, through the mouth, eventually making its way down to the intestines.

The path that science takes towards understanding the natural world is never straight and Landsteiner and Levaditi's early insights into how the poliovirus entered the body were not taken to their logical conclusion for several decades. The search to understand the mysteries of polio shifted across the Atlantic to the Rockefeller institute for Medical Sciences and its director, Simon Flexner. The institute had been founded by John D Rockefeller as the first biomedical institute in the United States. In Simon Flexner, it had an ambitious director and well-respected scientist who was eager to put the institute's resources to work tackling the major public health issues of the day.

Flexner was one of the foremost researchers of his day. He was particularly driven by the desire to make medicine more scientific, and to give clinical medicine a firm grounding based on work in the laboratory. He had first come to wider attention as a young researcher when he identified the bacteria behind a form of tropical dysentery. The discovery led to him having the bacteria named after him as *shigella flexneri*. Flexner's career continued to be marked by a string of achievements, both as a leader of medical research institutes and as a researcher. But one of his biggest failures was in his attempt to understand the way the poliovirus infected humans.

When news of Landsteiner's infection of monkeys reached the United States, Flexner was perfectly positioned to rise to the challenge of taking his work forward. The Rockefeller Institute had the resources to invest in monkeys as well as researchers, and polio had emerged as a major public health concern after an epidemic swept through New York in 1906. Flexner found that it was possible to transmit the disease between monkeys by injecting poliovirus into their brains and all his subsequent experimental work was based on infecting monkeys through the brain. He soon found he was able to infect monkeys through their nasal passages. This convinced him that this was how humans were getting infected, and that the virus passed from the nasal passage to the brain where it caused paralysis.

What Flexner did not see was that over the decades, after being constantly injected into monkey brains and replicating in monkey brain tissue, his laboratory viral strains had adapted to monkeys' nervous tissue. This meant they had begun to behave in ways that the natural poliovirus did not. The wild, or natural, poliovirus did not and could not pass directly from the nasal passages to the brains in humans.

But such was Flexner's reputation and his personality, that his findings became the prevalent dogma. Based on his theories, Flexner advised that children should have zinc sulphate rubbed into their nostrils to protect them from polio. Dorothy Horstmann, a well-known polio researcher at the Yale Medical School, later observed wryly that this resulted in the loss of sense of smell in some, but not in the prevention of poliomyelitis.[6]

There were clues that the poliovirus made its way to other parts of the body, and did not travel from nose to brain. A group of Swedish researchers had demonstrated in 1912 that the virus could be recovered from the small intestines of fatal and non-fatal polio cases, indicating that the virus might be entering the body through the mouth. But such was Flexner's dominance that it was only in the 1930s that polio research pulled itself out of a dead end, and began to understand the poliovirus and its route of infection a bit better.

In 1931, an outbreak of polio in New Haven drew the attention of two researchers at Yale Medical School: John Paul and James Trask. They set up the Poliomyelitis Study Unit at Yale, acquired some monkeys and set to work to try to understand the disease better. Their colleague Dorothy Horstmann wrote that the two researchers set themselves apart from other polio researchers by trying to isolate the virus from patients with mild forms of illness, much as researchers in Sweden had done twenty years earlier.

Paul and Trask found virus in the faeces of a polio patient, and also recovered infectious virus from sewage, an indication that the poliovirus travelled to the intestines, and was perhaps an intestinal infection.

It took another decade or so to establish that from the intestines, the virus passes into the blood stream—a condition known as viremia—before travelling to the central nervous system.

Once it was known that the poliovirus entered the blood stream, it became possible to think of protecting people from the disease by inducing antibodies in the blood through vaccination.

Creating a vaccine, and indeed a full understanding of the pathology of the virus would require another two decades of work. The development of molecular techniques enabled studies on the structure of the poliovirus, its inner workings, its method of infecting cells, and its relationship to other closely linked viruses, turning it into one of the most closely studied human pathogens.

* * *

All viruses are tiny, thousands of times smaller than the finest grain of salt and visible to the eye only through an electron microscope. The poliovirus is among the smallest of viruses, little more than a sparse set of genetic instructions on a sliver of RNA, covered in a protein coat for protection. The poliovirus genome is 7,400 nucleotide base pairs long with each pair of RNA molecules linked to a backbone of sugar and phosphate molecules. In contrast to the poliovirus, the genome of even the common E. coli bacteria is nearly 5 million nucleotides long, the mouse genome is 2.8 billion base pairs while the human genome has over 3.3 billion nucleotide base pairs.

Despite, or perhaps because of, its tiny size the poliovirus is an elegantly designed particle. Its outer coat, or capsid, is shaped as an icosahedron, a symmetrical twenty-sided structure arranged around twelve vertices. X-ray crystallography reveals a spherical virus with surface proteins that give it a bumpy cauliflower like surface. Tightly packed under this outer coat is the strand of RNA containing the poliovirus genome. Unlike higher forms of life, the poliovirus has its genetic information coded in RNA, rather than DNA. RNA is chemically less stable that DNA, and RNA-based based genetic replication is much more prone to errors than DNA-based based replication, since it does not have a mechanism to correct and eliminate errors when its genes are copied. But to get over these difficulties, RNA-based viruses tend to have small genomes and reproduce rapidly in the cell, producing large numbers of progeny so that even if all do not survive, large enough numbers will to ensure propagation.

Viruses lack the cellular mechanisms to reproduce; all they contain is a genetic code that needs to be inserted into a living cell so that the host cell's internal machinery can be hijacked to produce copies of the virus. In many cases so many copies of the virus are produced that the unfortunate host cell explodes, scattering viral particles which then infect other cells. In other cases, the process is less dramatic, and host cell and viral particles co-exist for a while before the viral particles exit to find new cells to infect.

The key to survival for a virus is to find the right host cell to infect. Viruses attach themselves to hosts by binding to specific molecules, or receptors on the surface of a cell. As the virologist Dorothy Crawford puts it, a cell receptor is like a lock, and only viruses that carry the correct receptor binding key to open the lock can enter a cell.[7] Even if a virus can enter a cell, it is not guaranteed that the cellular environment will be conducive to its replication. The virus needs to find a host cell that is both susceptible to infection because it has a suitable receptor, and permissive in the sense of having a cellular environment that supports viral replication. Over millions of years, viruses have adapted and evolved with host species, some able to infect multiple hosts, while other have adapted to single hosts.

Over the course of its evolution, the poliovirus has come to adapt to a single known host: man. Humans are the only known species to have cells with the receptors poliovirus needs to start an infection. A few old-world monkey species, including the rhesus and the cynomogolous, can be infected experimentally through injections with the poliovirus. Karl Landsteiner in Vienna was fortunate that he had these two species on hand when he tried to search for the infectious agent that caused polio, but they do not get infected through any natural route. It is possible that there are other non-human primates that are hosts of the poliovirus, but no evidence of this has been found so far.

The poliovirus is part of the picornavirus family (viral names are not particularly imaginative: picornavirus is a lexical amalgam of pico, or small, and rna virus). Within the sprawling picornavirus family, the poliovirus falls within a group of viruses known as human enteroviruses, which cause a variety of diseases in humans including

11

hand foot and mouth disease, acute conjunctivitis, and other polio-like paralytic diseases.

Poliovirus itself comes in three variations or serotypes: Type 1, Type 2 and Type 3, that are near identical except for slight differences in the loops of amino acids on the surface of the virus. These variations between the three types are important in the body's fight against polio. When someone gets infected with polio, the human immune system begins to generate antibodies that recognise sites on these loops on the poliovirus. Because each of the three types of poliovirus has minute differences in these loops, antibodies generated by the body after an infection by say Type 1, are not effective against the other two strains. To be fully protected against polio, the body needs to have all three types of antibodies in the blood. This in turn had implications when polio vaccines were developed: three vaccines had to be created to protect against the three strains of virus.

The life-cycle of a virus is driven by a single goal: to find a host cell to invade, to replicate in that cell and then find new cells for the progeny to infect. The symptoms that viral infections cause are often part of the virus' strategy to find new hosts. In the case of flu viruses, the coughs and sneezes that are typical symptoms are the route the virus uses to escape from the body of an infected person to find someone new to infect. The rhinovirus that causes common colds infects the cells that line the nose, causing the typical runny nose symptoms, and spreads to fresh hosts when infected people touch their noses and spread the virus through their hands by touching others.

The poliovirus can only infect human cells that contain a protein on their surface known as CD 155 that is found in different forms on cells in various parts of the body. These are found in the mucosal layers in the throat and pharynx, and in the Peyer's patches of the small intestine and in lymph nodes around the small intestine.

The poliovirus journey to infection begins when it enters the human body through the mouth, as a lifeless, inert set of chemicals. These minute viral particles are hardy enough to survive the first lines of defence that the body throws up to invaders entering through the mouth (the saliva in the mouth and the gastric acid in the stomach). Some viral particles begin to replicate in the pharynx, but the majority pass through the duodenum into the relatively more benign environment of the small intestines. As they are propelled through the twists and turns of the intestine, some viral particles will bump against cells with CD 155.

Like a drowning man being swept along by a raging river clutching a passing tree trunk, the poliovirus manages to latch onto a strand of CD 155, at which point biochemical forces at the molecular level come to play. The poliovirus has narrow, canyon shaped depressions along some of its sides, perfectly shaped and biochemically receptive to locking onto CD 155. The slender CD 155 molecule pushes into the viral canyon, and triggers a process that causes the protein coating of the virus to unlock, turning a set of inert chemicals into a self-replicating pathogen.

The exact steps by which the poliovirus penetrates a cell after it latches onto its receptor are still not completely understood. But one hypothesis is that the poliovirus uses a protein to punch little holes into the membrane of the host cells, through which it injects its RNA into the cell. Once the cell membrane is pierced and viral particles enter into the cytoplasm of the cell, they encounter a new and hazardous environment of cellular enzymes and chemicals that can destroy the poliovirus RNA. To survive this, the poliovirus has a mechanism that rapidly takes charge of a cell's machinery to turn it into a virus-making factory. The virus' RNA serves as messenger RNA which the host cell's ribosomes, or protein-manufacturing machine, uses to create the proteins that make the poliovirus.

At first, large polyproteins are created which are then cut by enzymes into the proteins that will eventually make up the coat of the virus. The virus takes over small parts of the host cell to create a micro-environment in which its own RNA can be replicated. Enzymes are also released that prevent the host cell from using its own protein-synthesising machinery, reserving it for the use of the virus. The new RNA and the capsule proteins come together to create new poliovirus particles, and within an estimated seven or eight hours the host cell is literally stuffed full of new poliovirus particles. The cell host dies under this burden releasing new viral particles into the environment, which in turn look for fresh cells to infect.

Life at the viral level is a game of numbers: researchers estimate that only around 1 per cent of viral particles released this way will find fresh cells to infect in the same host. Some find neighbouring cells, while others pass through the intestines and are ejected into the wider environment through the faeces. The poliovirus ability to find fresh hosts once it is outside the human body, wrapped in faeces, depends on the external environment. The virus needs to enter a new human host through the mouth. This is most likely to happen in environments where faecal contamination of drinking water is common because sewage and water can mix, or when hygiene is poor and that faecal matter can pass from hands to mouth.

It is one of nature's myriad paradoxes that the paralysis caused by the poliovirus is almost accidental, and completely unnecessary to the virus survival. All the poliovirus needs to replicate and propagate itself is to gain access to cells with CD 4 receptors in the intestines and pharynx. Occasionally though, the polioviruses makes its way to the nerve cells of the spinal column, where it causes paralysis. Creeping into the spinal column is a rare, and largely inexplicable event for the poliovirus, and only between 1 in 100 to 1 in 1,000 cases of polio infection result in paralysis. Most infections cause no symptoms at all, or mild symptoms of a fever and sore throat that pass in a few days. As the polio virologist Vincent Racaniello wrote 'the infamous propensity of the poliovirus to invade the central nervous system and specifically target motor neurons is rare and accidental and it is neither a prerequisite nor does it present a benefit for its normal life cycle in humans...'.[8]

The mechanisms by which a gut virus like the poliovirus finds its way to the central nervous system is not entirely clear. It is generally accepted that the poliovirus initially replicates in the mucosal cells of the pharynx and small intestine and passes into the blood through the lymph nodes. In most cases, the immune system clears the virus out of the body at this stage, and the disease proceeds no further, and no symptoms are felt. In around 4–8 per cent of cases, the disease goes to a second stage, known as abortive poliomyelitis. Here the virus continues to replicate in the body and enters the blood stream for a second time, producing a range of symptoms including sore throat, fever, abdominal discomfort and a general feeling of malaise. In the vast majority of these cases, the disease ends there. In about 1 to 2 per cent of cases where the disease goes to this second stage, the poliovirus enters the central nervous system, attacks nerve cells of the spinal cord, and causes paralysis.

Different researchers experimenting on mice have all concluded that the virus enters a peripheral nerve at a junction between nerve and muscle. After this it travels along the axons, the long fibres that extend out of every nerve cell, until it reaches the nucleus of the neuron or nerve cell in the spinal cord. Other studies using lab mice indicate that the virus can be carried by the blood stream to the brain.

By whatever method it travels, the poliovirus attacks the nerve cells of the anterior grey column of the spinal cord, which contain the neurons responsible for controlling muscles of the limbs. This causes the paralysis that characterises polio. In around one fifth of paralytic cases, the virus attacks the nerves of the cervical area of the spinal cord, which controls the diaphragm and breathing, and patients have to be put on mechanical ventilators until they recover some of their nerve and muscle functions. In a small fraction of cases, the virus destroys nerves in the bulbar region of the brain, causing a variety of symptoms including difficulties in breathing and facial paralysis.

* * *

The poliovirus has infected human beings since the earliest times; the mild and often symptomless disease that most poliovirus infections cause indicate a virus that has long been habituated to its human host. Virologists who study the evolving relationship between virus and hosts, suggest that the severity of disease caused by a virus is the greatest when the virus is first introduced to a new host. For example, when measles and smallpox were introduced by European conquerors and settlers to native populations in the Americas and Australia the effect on local people who had never encountered these viruses before, was devastating. In the sixteenth century, measles brought to the New World by the Spanish conquistadores is believed to have triggered epidemics that killed around 50 per cent of the population of present day Honduras. In Europeans who had been long exposed to these pathogens and whose immune systems had encountered them at an early age, the disease symptom were often milder, and epidemics were rare.

This mutual accommodation between virus and host is beneficial to both. As the medical historian William McNeill puts it, 'A disease organism that kills its host quickly creates a crisis for itself, since a new host must somehow be found often enough, and soon enough, to keep its own chains of generation going. ...Optimal conditions for host and parasite occur, often though not necessarily always, when each continue to live in the other's presence for an indefinite period of time with no very significant diminution of normal activity on either side.'[9] For centuries, the poliovirus and humans appeared to have existed in equilibrium, with the virus causing largely mild or symptomless infection and occasional cases of paralysis.

But towards the late nineteenth century, in the wealthier parts of the world, something happened to disturb this equilibrium. As we have seen, beginning around 1880, outbreaks of paralytic disease were reported first in Sweden and Norway then in the United States and other parts of Europe. The outbreaks in Scandinavia appeared as clusters of cases of children, mostly under the age of six, who developed fever followed by paralysis of the limbs. Several outbreaks were recorded in the last two decades of the century, all occurring in the summer in isolated rural communities, and targeting children under the age of 5 or 6. In 1905, Sweden and Norway recorded the largest epidemics of polio that had been recorded to date, with around 1,000 cases in each country. Unlike previous years, the cases were not confined to pockets of rural communities, but occurred across both countries.

In 1894, the first major outbreak was recorded in the United States in Rutland County, Vermont, where there were 132 cases of polio among adolescents as well as young children. Outbreaks of poliomyelitis were to become increasingly common in the United States, involving larger numbers of cases. In 1916, an outbreak in New York city recorded 9,000 cases of paralysis, many of them in the older age groups. Summer epidemics of polio would rage across the Western world in the first half of the twentieth century, raising two intriguing questions. The first was why a disease that had never been known to take epidemic form was suddenly exploding in this way. Second—in a reversal of expectations—why were wealthy parts of the world with high standards of hygiene and health care being affected, not the poorer, less developed parts of the world with worse systems of sanitation and hygiene.

The answers to these questions indicate the occasionally counterintuitive impact that economic, social and cultural changes can have on the relationship between man and microbe. In societies with poorer sanitation, the poliovirus is endemic and widely prevalent in the environment. As a result, children come into contact with the virus at a very early age, often shortly after birth. Since only between 1 in a 100 to 1 in 1,000 infections lead to paralysis, most children develop mild or asymptomatic infections that cause no harm, and are then protected for life. A small proportion of infected children develops paralysis. Through this early exposure to the virus a large proportion of the population develops lifelong immunity, and so there are never a sufficient number of unexposed people for an epidemic to develop.

But as hygiene and general living conditions improved, the numbers of children exposed to the poliovirus declined and so correspondingly did population immunity. The pool of children and young adults who had no immunity to polio increased, allowing explosive outbreaks to spread. As one work on the history of polio describes it 'with increasing economic development and correspondingly improved resources for community and household hygiene, and with the additional advantage of a temperate zone climate, the opportunities for immunising infections among infants and young children were reduced…the delay in exposure increased the pool of susceptibles opening the way for rapid and explosive spread of the virus once they did enter the population, in contrast to the steady, endemic transmission of the preceding phase.'[10]

The large number of paralytic cases during these epidemics was explained by the fact that children were getting exposed to the poliovirus later in life, sometimes as young adults. The chances of polio infections leading to paralysis increased with age.

So rare were reports of polio from developing tropical countries, that for most of the first half of the last century, it was widely considered to be a disease of temperate climes. Occasional surveys of lameness and sporadic clinical reports indicated there was polio in these countries. But because so many had been exposed to the virus at a young age and developed immunity, there were few cases of paralytic disease.

The extent to which the poliovirus was present in tropical countries was only recognised during the Second World War. US and British soldiers stationed in theatres of war in Asia and the Middle East, began contracting polio, even though the local population showed no signs of disease. Cases were reported among British and New Zealand soldiers in Egypt and India, and US soldiers in the Philippines. US forces landed in

Leyte in the Philippines in October 1944, and the first soldier came down with polio sixteen days later. By the end of the year, thirty-nine cases among US troops were reported of which fourteen were fatal. There were no reported cases among local people. Albert Sabin, who was a doctor in the US Army Medical Corps during the war and would later develop the oral polio vaccine, investigated polio among US troops. He concluded that the virus was transmitting endemically among the local population even though they showed no sign of disease.

To the epidemiologist, time, place and person are the questions that need to be answered when trying to understand a disease. Who are the kind of people being infected? Are there patterns to be found in the ages of the people being infected, their gender, their economic status? Are there clues to be found in the geographical locations where people are falling ill? Are there patterns to be found in the time of year, or seasons during which people tend to get infected? By seeking answers to these basic questions, epidemiologists try and understand the nature of disease, its routes of transmission, and which places and people are most likely to be vulnerable.

These epidemiological variables of time, place and person are useful not only to understand a disease, but also how different societies respond to a disease. When Spanish conquistadores brought smallpox and measles to the new world, the tragedy that ensued could have been predicted by understanding the nature of the society that was being invaded by the disease (and the humans who brought the disease). These were societies that were sophisticated in many ways but did not have a modern understanding of disease, or ways to reduce its impact. So, when the Aztecs of Mexico were stricken by smallpox after contact with the Spanish conquistador Hernando Cortez, their society collapsed, both physically and psychologically. As William McNeill writes, the Aztecs would have noted that this disease killed the Aztecs, but left the Spaniards unharmed. The only explanation for this was that the gods of the Spaniards was superior to the gods of the Aztecs, and that surrender was the only option. 'The religions, priesthoods and way of life built around the old Indian gods could not survive such a demonstration of the superior power of the God the Spaniards worshipped. Little wonder, then, that the Indians accepted Christianity and surrendered to Spanish control so meekly. God had shown Himself on their side, and each new outbreak of infectious disease imported from Europe (and soon from Africa as well) renewed the lesson.'[11]

Smallpox hastened the collapse of Aztec society because the Aztecs were unable to understand or respond to this pathogen. It happened at a time in human society when Europe was the centre of global power, European colonialism was expanding and it was regarded as natural that more powerful societies would exploit weaker ones. Therefore, there were no global efforts, as might have happened in our times, to rush aid and resources to the Aztecs to fight the disease.

When the poliovirus caused epidemics in the late nineteenth and twentieth centuries, the time, place and persons it hit were very different, and so was the response. The virus was attacking the most economically and scientifically advanced societies in the world, societies that would fight back and protect themselves by first understanding the disease, and then finding ways to thwart the virus. The poliovirus had survived and coexisted with humans through the centuries. But the epidemics that rocked the Western world marked a turning point in the relationship between humans and polio. They hit the United States, the wealthiest and most scientifically advanced country in the world, homing in on its suburban middle-class children. This set in train a set of events that would eventually lead to a global campaign to wipe the virus off the face of the earth.

Had polio been a disease that targeted the poorer countries of the world in African and Asia, it is unlikely that the long, expensive process to understand it, produce vaccines, and eventually eradicate the virus would have acquired such momentum. And had the United States not been hit by repeated epidemics, it is far from certain that a global campaign to eradicate the virus would have got off the ground.

2

THE PRESIDENT AND THE POLIOVIRUS

On the morning of 11 August 1921, Franklin Delano Roosevelt awoke at his summer home on Campobello Island, off the coast of Maine, feverish, in pain, and with a weakness in his left leg. Roosevelt was 39 years old, and at the early stages of a political career that would eventually lead to the presidency of the United States.

The previous day had been a typically frenetic vacation day for the Roosevelt family. Accompanied by his five children and his wife Eleanor, FDR had taken his boat out for a sail in the Bay of Fundy, and noticed a brush fire on a small island nearby. He and the children stopped to fight the fire with pine boughs and spent several hot exhausting hours until it was extinguished. After they returned, they decided they needed an afternoon swim, and ran over three kilometres to a pond on the other side of the island where they splashed around. Then they rounded off the day's activity with a plunge in the cold waters of the bay, and a run back home.

Roosevelt was feeling unusually tired when he got back, and thought he was catching a chill. He retired to bed but had trouble sleeping, and was cold despite his heavy blankets. The next morning, when he tried to stand, his left leg collapsed under him. He also had a high fever. A local doctor who was summoned, thought it was just a bad cold, but Roosevelt's symptoms worsened.

A day later he was paralysed from the chest down, and in excruciating pain.

A surgeon who happened to be holidaying close by was called in, and after an examination decided Roosevelt was suffering from a blood clot in the lower spinal cord, and prescribed massages to move the clot. The massages were painful, and did nothing to relieve the paralysis. Soon his hands and arms became paralysed as well. He lost control over his bodily functions and needed a catheter and enemas. His body ached constantly and even the slightest touch on his skin was painful. The Roosevelt clan then contacted Robert Lovett, a professor of surgery at Harvard, and an authority on polio, or infantile paralysis as it was known. Dr Lovett examined Roosevelt on 25 August and declared there was no doubt that the patient had polio.

Lovett's diagnosis came as a shock. Most victims of polio were young children, or teenagers, and adult cases of the disease were unusual. There is a continuing debate on whether Roosevelt actually suffered from polio, or whether he was stricken by Guillaume Barré syndrome, a neurological disorder. Armond Goldman and his colleagues at the Department of Pediatrics at the University of Texas Medical School in Galveston, have strongly argued the latter case. They say that FDR's age, the paralysis on both sides of the body that ascended from his legs to his arms and upper body, as well as the numbness, the pain on touch and the bladder and bowel dysfunction indicated Guillaume Barré syndrome.[1] Others maintain the polio diagnosis was correct, and surmise that he might have been infected when he attended a boy scout event a couple of days earlier.[2] Since laboratory tests that would definitively indicate polio were not conducted, we will never know.

But it is almost irrelevant whether he was stricken by the poliovirus or whether there was another cause for his condition. What is important in the wider context of how humans understand and battle with disease, was that Roosevelt, and everyone else around him believed he had polio. This in turn played a pivotal role in how the United States came to perceive polio. More importantly, Roosevelt's political and social prominence led to the creation of a private foundation that would raise unprecedented amounts of money to rehabilitate polio patients, and fund research that would eventually result in the production of vaccines to eliminate the disease.

Roosevelt had a profound impact on the way the American public perceived polio. Earlier, polio was seen as a life-long sentence to being confined to wheel chairs and crutches, staying largely indoors, being viewed as an object of pity and unable to lead a productive life. Roosevelt helped build the idea that it was possible to triumph over the disease.[3]

Part of the triumph in Roosevelt's case was illusory. He remained wheelchair bound for the rest of his life, never regained the use of his legs, and was unable to walk, or even stand, without the use of heavy metal braces concealed under his clothing. Yet there are only rare photographs of him in a wheelchair. A complicit press helped the President hide from the public the fact that he never regained the use of his legs after being stricken. The historian of polio in the United States, David Oshinsky writes, 'He [Roosevelt] reached a gentleman's agreement with the press not to be photographed in a wheelchair or in a helpless position. He hid his leg braces under long capes and blankets. The Secret Service prepared for his speaking appearances by constructing portable ramps and putting hand grips on the podium.'[4]

Roosevelt's 'splendid deception', as Hugh Gallagher, one of his biographers, has termed it, helped him win the presidency of the United States four times, but also helped transform the narrative around polio in the United States. It went from being a disease characterised by people on crutches and wheelchairs, to one that could be overcome. The image of the ever-smiling Roosevelt, his cigarette holder perched at a jaunty angle in his mouth with no hint that he was in any way disabled, told Americans that polio could be fought and defeated.

Roosevelt also determined the course of how America and the world responded to polio by throwing his considerable political influence behind a private foundation he created. The National Foundation for Infantile Paralysis (NFIP) would raise unprecedently large sums of money to fund a decades' long programme of research. This would eventually lead to not one, but two polio vaccines, that would end the fear of polio in the United States and the rest of the world. It would also make it possible to eradicate the disease globally.

The money was raised in a uniquely American way, with donations from ordinary people, channelled into a foundation which in turn set priorities and funded researchers in universities on a scale never seen before. Research teams and laboratories such as Jonas Salk's at the University of Pittsburgh and Albert Sabin's at the University of Cincinnati were generously funded by the NFIP for decades. The US government and health service had virtually no role in the fight against polio. The NFIP has been described as 'one of the most successful voluntary organisations in history, second only to the American Red Cross in the sheer volume of dollars it was able to attract every year...In its heyday in the early 1950s, the privately supported and administered NFIP spent ten times as much on polio research as the tax-supported National Institutes of Health.'[5]

To help fundraising, the NFIP had a sophisticated publicity department, with script writers, photographers and journalists churning out a steady stream of material that helped to ensure that polio was never forgotten. This was even in the midst of other crises besetting America, first the Great Depression, and then the Second World War. Jane Smith in her book on the development of the Salk polio vaccine writes about the generation of propaganda for the campaign. 'The Radio and Film department,' she says, 'later expanded to include television, churned out dramatic scripts about the heroic people who struggled against the terrors of polio, the dedicated doctors and scientists who worked to help them, and the generous citizens who made it all possible. Reports of scientific 'breakthroughs' were placed in popular magazines like *Reader's Digest*, and gossip columnists were fed items about movie stars filming appeals for the March of Dimes and socialites collecting change on corners.'[6]

Polio was a terrible disease, one that any parent or child would dread. But the prominence it received in the public mind was also heightened by the publicity given to the disease by the NFIP, the institution Roosevelt helped launch. The NFIP led the fight against polio by raising funds on a scale that was unprecedented for rehabilitation and research. But fundraising depended on keeping polio in the public eye. Dr John Paul, the author of a comprehensive scientific history of polio, wrote that in its early years, the NFIP 'seemed to place more emphasis on promoting the spectre of paralytic poliomyelitis and on fund raising activities than on anything else.' As Daniel Wilson writes 'the use of poster children by the NFIP to raise funds kept the image of the crippled polio survivor before the public, even though many of those initially paralysed were left with minor deformities.'[7] David Oshinsky observes, 'Rarely, if ever had Americans been exposed to so much information about a single disease. Most of it came from the NFIP which skilfully mixed the public's dread of polio with its larger message of inevitable triumph.' Articles about polio in magazines, particularly those targeted at women were ubiquitous, and much of this material was commissioned and often ghost written by the NFIP's publicity team.

The publicity machine turned polio into an ever-present enemy that needed to be fought and defeated. Meanwhile the reliance on small donations by ordinary people, and recruitment of a volunteer army to collect dimes and organise fund raising events gave people a stake in the battle.[8]

The attack on Pearl Harbour and the United States entry into the Second World War made the Foundation worry about whether it would be proper to continue to focus public attention on polio in the midst of a larger national crisis. Other war-related appeals were being made to the public to contribute to war bonds and to the Red Cross. Roosevelt however was clear that fundraising for polio needed to continue. 'The fight being waged against infantile paralysis... is an essential part of the struggle in which we are all engaged. Nothing is closer to my heart than the health of our boys and girls and young men and women. To me it is one of the front lines of our National Defense.'[9]

It helped the NFIP's fundraising that the war years also saw a steady rise in the number of cases of polio, from around 9,000 in 1944, to more than 19,000 in 1944. This rise in polio continued after the war, peaking at around 58,000 cases in 1952. The surge in polio cases among babies born during the post-war baby boom to parents who had experienced the war, and were looking forward to raising families in peace and prosperity of post war America, added to the national anxiety over polio. It also increased the urgency for finding a way to prevent and stamp out this crippler of the nation's children. Jane Smith observes, 'The unprecedented surge in the birth rate, and the new national interest in the care and protection of children made the goals of the NFIP seem more worthy and more urgent than ever. More people were having more babies, and there is nothing like becoming a parent to focus your attention on a childhood disease.'[10] Money poured into the NFIP, as did public expectation that a cure, or a vaccine for the disease be found. Polio was also terrifying because it struck at a time when most infectious diseases were on the wane as a result of simple measures such as near universal access to clean drinking water, indoor plumbing and more hygienic living conditions. A graph of the death rates from infectious diseases in the United States, shows a steady fall from around 1900 (the only blip being the deaths from the influenza pandemic of 1919).

Cleanliness, and an obsession with germs, was also becoming a feature of middle-class America. The discoveries of Robert Koch and Louis Pasteur fuelled the anxiety that pathogens were the causes of infectious diseases. A jump in literacy had quadrupled the numbers of magazines in the United States, and cleanliness, hygiene and the problems posed by germs were a staple of the articles they contained. 'Disease from Public Laundries', and 'The Perilous Barbershop' were typical topics, and articles contained advice such as fumigating your home each time a guest departed, or spraying cyanide to destroy germs. This particular procedure involved running rapidly from room to room and instantly closing the door once the spray had been deployed.[11] Paper money, and even books borrowed from public libraries were seen as hidden spreaders of lethal germs.

These warnings of the dangers posed by microbes were reflected in changes in personal hygiene and social habits. Men shaved their beards and women shortened their skirts to avoid trapping germs, while people began to cover their coughs and sneezes. Sales of soap and other products offering protection from germs soared. But none of this seemed to be able to stop the poliovirus.

Ironically, better standards of hygiene and access to safe water were probably the reasons why polio emerged in epidemic form. The scientific consensus is that these epidemics were caused as hygiene improved because infants were no longer being exposed to the poliovirus at a young age. Polio virologists Neal Nathanson and Olen Kew, write that in earlier times, when the poliovirus was endemic, most infants were probably infected within their first six to twelve months, at a time when they had immunity from their nursing mothers. This maternally-derived immunity meant that the poliovirus could still infect their guts, causing at worst mild stomach symptoms. But it was unable to get into the child's blood stream to cause paralysis. This early, symptomless infection provided immunity for the rest of the person's life. However, better hygiene and improved sanitation meant that children came into contact with the poliovirus at a later age, when they were no longer protected by their mothers' antibodies. They point out that the earliest epidemics occurred in countries like Sweden where hygiene and sanitation were the most advanced. As public health improved in other countries, a similar pattern followed with epidemics of polio breaking out.[12]

Though polio is an enteric virus, and is transmitted through the faecal-oral route, the poliovirus also infects the pharynx. In countries with better sanitation it is thought that the virus is passed person to person through respiratory droplets, rather than through contamination by faeces. The fact that cleanliness did not seem to lessen the chance of infection was part of the terror the disease caused in the United States. The only thing that it seemed parents could do was keep their children at home during the summer months and so children were prohibited from going to swimming pools, playgrounds or movie theatres for fear of catching polio.

Those who did catch the disease underwent months of painful physical therapy at the end of which they might or might not regain full use of their limbs. Children who developed bulbar polio (which develops when the virus attacks the nerves in the spinal cord that control breathing) were often confined to enormous mechanical ventilators known as iron lungs for weeks, months and years, until they either recovered, or died.

Polio was not the most serious disease that affected Americans during the last century. Scarlet fever, tuberculosis, whooping cough and measles had a higher incidence than polio, but polio provoked a unique dread. This was because it affected children and it appeared to strike almost at random (this appearance of randomness was because most of those infected with the virus showed no symptoms, and only the rare case developed paralysis). Even in the case of those who developed paralysis, there was no telling who would be left with only mild paralysis, who would be crippled for life, and who would die of the disease.

The historian of polio (and polio sufferer), Daniel Wilson observes that the fear of polio could approach hysteria during epidemic years but was often driven as much by cultural and social factors as by the reality of the disease itself. This was a disease that seemed to strike at the very heart of what it meant to be American. 'Many parents feared that polio, along with two other post war specters, communism and nuclear war, threatened their chance to achieve the American dream...'

he writes. 'Because the American dream envisioned only healthy children, not ones wearing braces and using wheel chairs.'[13]

Wilson also draws an interesting parallel between these epidemics of polio hitting at the heart of the American dream, and the other threat to the American dream, the Cold War with the Soviet Union. The stealthy way in which polio crept through communities to strike random individuals, seemed almost like an act of subversion. 'Thus the polio epidemics at mid-century bore a striking similarity to the concurrent cold war fears of Communist subversion, in which convicted spies were seen as only the visible tip of a vast, hidden conspiracy.'

Both the nature of the disease, as well as the publicity given to it, resulted in polio occupying a place in American minds that no other disease did. It seemed to threaten the country's future by crippling children, a disease that seemed impervious to all the amenities in hygiene and sanitation that the middle classes of one of the richest and most advanced societies in the world enjoyed. Polio seemed to mock the American dream.

This heightened perception of polio as a unique threat to society was not shared in other parts of the world. In the poorer parts of the world polio crippled children at a rate that was perhaps equal to the United States, but it was seen as just another disease among a rich landscape of infectious diseases. Polio was endemic in the developing world, and most children were exposed to the disease early in life, and developed lifelong immunity. Between one in every 100 and one in every 1,000 children infected by the poliovirus developed paralysis. So, it was not uncommon to see children crippled by polio. But polio was just one among a raft of infectious diseases that children and adults suffered from, most of which had higher rates of morbidity and mortality. By the second half of the twentieth century, as sanitation and general health conditions improved, countries in the developing world began to see epidemics of polio, just as the United States and Western Europe had. But polio was never regarded as an exceptionally dreadful disease in the way it was in the United States.

Even in Western Europe, which also suffered epidemics of polio in the last century, the disease was not seen as a uniquely dangerous threat. Tony Gould, the British author and journalist, recounts that though children were crippled in the United Kingdom, 'there was never the same kind of urgency about polio; it was a comparatively rare disease, with only local and small-scale epidemics, until after the Second World War, and—partly for that reason—there was no pressure group comparable to the NFIP.'[14]

Scandinavia, and Sweden in particular, was as badly, if not worse hit, by polio as the United States. One estimate has it that the incidence of polio in Sweden, in relation to its small population was higher than the US and Canada. Polio struck fear among Scandinavian parents, just as in the United States, and was regarded as a serious public health problem in epidemic years. But it was not perceived as it was in the United States, as a uniquely important threat, that required a national effort to conquer if the American dream was to be preserved.

This perception of polio in the United States would have a global impact. By the end of the Second World War, the United States had emerged on top of the global hierarchy of nations, the richest, and the most powerful country in the post-war world. The advantage of being the most powerful country on earth, is the influence it provides in setting the global agenda: deciding which issues are important and which are not. Polio was a major disease threat to Americans, and this perception spilled onto the global stage and made a campaign to eradicate the disease an almost natural thing to do. It was assumed that other countries, particularly developing countries, saw polio in the same light that the United States and Western Europe did, and would pay the same attention to it. But this was not the case.

The American experience of polio is essential to understanding how the GPEI developed, as well as the problems the eradication campaign would encounter in the many countries which had experienced polio differently from the Western world. The sociologist Jeremy Shiffman writes 'global polio eradication has been positioned as a humanitarian crusade to rid the world of a scourge that has afflicted children for millennia. Many older advocates from industrialised nations may view this positioning as both credible, accepting the idea that polio is truly a problem the world can be rid of, and salient, remembering a time when polio caused havoc each year in their own countries.'[15] In the developing world however, people were more likely to question why, among all the diseases that they were afflicted with, polio was being given such great prominence. They were likely to ask, as Sabiu, the farmer in Marke village in Kano in northern Nigeria, did, 'Why this polio, polio all the time?'

* * *

In addition to giving the disease salience, the US experience, and particularly the way the NFIP led the fight influenced the way the Global Polio Eradication Initiative would operate under the WHO.

The Global Polio Eradication Initiative was the first example of private organisations getting involved at a global level to control disease. Rotary, a private service organisation of businessmen and other professionals along with the WHO, UNICEF (the UN children's organisation) and the US Centers for Disease Control (CDC) led the eradication campaign. In 2008, the Bill and Melinda Gates Foundation joined the original polio eradication partners, creating a unique coalition of a private foundation, a private service organisation, two inter-governmental organisations (WHO and UNICEF) and a US government organisation (the CDC). Once the Gates Foundation came on board, private money from Gates and Rotary became important drivers of the programme, and along with other private philanthropic contributions made up roughly half the GPEI's annual funding in most years.

Though the polio eradication programme was ultimately responsible to governments, the extensive private money also made them autonomous from governments in the countries they worked in. Bill Gates' involvement in the campaign allowed him to pick up the phone and lobby heads of government and heads of state to push polio eradication in their countries. In many of the less developed countries, the GPEI also bypassed national health services, and directly ran vaccination campaigns, paying vaccinators, and supervising their work. The NFIP too worked independently of the US health services in deciding what research it would fund, and how it would conduct its rehabilitation work for polio victims. The only involvement of the government was when safety and ethical regulations needed to be met for vaccine trials and vaccine licensing.

The idea of a powerful private foundation working outside the government health machinery was not seen as unusual in the United States. It has had a strong tradition of private enterprise in areas that would otherwise be thought of as the preserve of the government. But at the global level, it was a mixed blessing. On the one hand, it gave the GPEI freedom and autonomy to work the way it wanted to. On the other hand, it separated polio from other government health services, and made it appear as an international programme in which local people had little interest or stake.

Probably the most striking similarity between the NFIP and the global eradication initiative, is its use of publicity and communication to shape the public narrative around polio. The NFIP's publicity department transformed polio from being not just a terrible disease, but the most dangerous disease threat the American public faced.

The GPEI too portrayed polio as a major threat that governments had to stamp out. Whatever other crises a country might face, the fight against polio had to continue, (as the NFIP argued during the Second World War). Whatever other diseases a country might be battling, fighting polio was the most urgent need of the day. In the midst of conflict, in the midst of famine, in the midst of civil war, the battle against polio had to continue. Thus, the WHO's member countries in 2012 urged polio-infected countries to declare polio a health emergency and implement emergency action plans. This was at a time when there were far more serious disease threats that were taking children's lives and were not declared an emergency. Two years later, polio was declared a public health emergency of international concern under the International Health Regulations. The global cases of polio ranged from 223 in 2012 to 359 in 2014, minuscule compared to other diseases. But the polio eradication campaign successfully kept the disease on the global health agenda, and lobbied governments with polio cases to take action, arguing that polio could make a global resurgence unless it was permanently stamped out.

The concept of community involvement in the fight against disease, pioneered by the NFIP in the United States, also found its echo in the global campaign against polio, through the involvement of Rotary. As we shall see in a later chapter, Rotary's involvement was crucial to the launching of the eradication campaign. It was Rotary club money, raised by its members from communities all over the world, that paid the salaries of the first WHO staff members hired to manage the global eradication programme. Rotarians across the world in the United States as well as India, Pakistan and Nigeria, would raise funds for the eradication campaign and volunteer for vaccination campaigns, organising community events just as the volunteers of the NFIP did.

Rotary's decision to get involved in global polio eradication began with US Rotarians, all of whom were familiar with the work of the NFIP. Rotarians in the United States, in their individual capacity and through clubs already had a history of involvement in raising funds for rehabilitating disabled children.[16] These same practices were emulated by Rotary clubs in other parts of the world, using similar strategies to the NFIP. Communal fund-raising events ranged from charity sales to bike-a-thons and walk-a-thons, as well as campaigns with celebrity endorsements.

But perhaps the greatest legacy the NFIP gave to the global eradication campaign were the two vaccines that it funded and helped develop. This is the story that I investigate in the next chapter.

3

THE SALK VACCINE

ENDING THE TERROR OF POLIO

Vaccines are generally acknowledged to be one of the greatest inventions of medical science. They are credited with saving more lives than penicillin, antibiotics, open heart surgery, kidney transplants or any other major innovations of modern medicine. Less than 100 years ago, whooping cough, measles, smallpox, and rubella were killers that people feared. Today, in the developed world and increasingly in the developing world, most children are vaccinated against these and other once common infectious diseases. Many doctors can spend their careers without seeing a case of whooping cough or meningitis. Vaccines are the tamers of infectious disease, and whenever new, dangerous, diseases such as HIV/AIDS or Ebola emerge, the first instinct of medical science is to try and develop a vaccine.

The development of two polio vaccines in the United States in the 1950s were essential stepping stones to eradication. Jonas Salk's killed virus vaccine, and Albert Sabin's live attenuated virus vaccine worked in different ways to produce immunity in the human body. Both had formidable strengths, as well as weaknesses. The Sabin vaccine was used through most of the global polio eradication campaign, but the Salk vaccine was brought in at the crucial final stages of the polio eradication campaign. The global polio eradication effort is a tale of two vaccines. The characteristics of these two vaccines, as well as the characters of the two men who produced them are part of the story of how the world decided to eradicate polio.

When polio scythed thorough the United States in the first half of the twentieth century, a vaccine was seen as the Holy Grail to protect against the disease. But so little was known about the virus, how it spread from person to person, and its behaviour in the human body, that creating a safe vaccine took decades of scientific effort. The road to success was marked by some spectacular failures.

The 1920s (when epidemics of polio became a regular occurrence in the United States) was in many ways a golden age for vaccine development. Between 1923 and 1927 vaccines were created for diphtheria, tuberculosis, tetanus and whooping cough.

Polio was different. In the early decades of the last century it was still a mysterious disease. Karl Landsteiner in Vienna had established it was caused by a virus, but beyond that little was known about how it transmitted from person to person, or even how it entered the human body and caused paralysis. Though little was known about the poliovirus, there were reasons to believe a vaccine could be effective against the disease. No one ever seemed to get polio twice, which meant that infection conferred life-long protection. If this was the case, it made sense to try and find ways to artificially induce immunity through a vaccine.

Researchers had begun experimenting with monkeys, injecting them under the skin with small amounts of poliovirus, and if they survived, injecting poliovirus directly into the brain, in quantities that would normally be guaranteed to paralyse the monkey. But monkeys that had been injected earlier with small doses of the virus under the skin, appeared to resist paralysis when they received a full dose of virus in the brain. This indicated that the first injection had triggered an immune response that protected the monkey from a second, more severe infection.

But the results from different labs were not always consistent, and even when the results were hopeful, there was no way to translate them into a vaccine that could be safely tested on humans. The ground-up suspension of polio-infected spinal cords that were used to immunise monkeys were far too dangerous to try on humans. So researchers began to try and kill, or inactivate the virus first, and see if the killed virus would stimulate an immune response.

Vaccines for bacterial diseases such as typhoid, the plague and cholera used killed bacteria. But this had never been tried for viral diseases like polio. Early vaccines for typhoid and cholera used bacteria that had been killed by heat and then injected into humans. The killed bacteria caused no disease, but provoked antibodies in the blood that could protect against future disease. But this did not work for polio: killing the virus with heat did not produce any immunity. Others tried killing the virus with formalin, but failed to produce anything safe enough, or effective enough in monkeys to use as a potential vaccine.

Safety was a big concern. When a mass of poliovirus was treated with formalin, it killed a substantial portion of the viral particles. But there was no guarantee that all the viral particles had been killed, and the consequence of a vaccine that could cause paralysis because it still contained some live viral material was too dangerous to consider.

These halting scientific efforts in the 1930s to work on monkeys to understand the different options for vaccine creation came to a disastrous end. Two sets of researchers working independently, Maurice Brodie and William Park at New York University, and John Kolmer at the Research Institute for Cutaneous Medicine at Philadelphia, tried vaccines on humans that had been barely tested and were potentially lethal. Brodie and Park developed an inactivated vaccine after grinding the spinal cords of monkeys infected with polio into an emulsion, and filtering it to remove impurities, before treating the mixture with formalin to kill the virus. They injected this mixture into twenty monkeys, all of which developed antibodies in their blood to polio, but suffered no apparent paralysis from the injection. Based on these very preliminary experiments on monkeys, Brodie and Park pushed ahead with trials on humans.

No one knew how safe the vaccine was. Had all the virus in the vaccine been completely killed, or was there enough live virus still left to cause polio in children? Beyond this were there other impurities in the vaccine that could cause side effects?

Brodie and Park first tested their crude vaccine on a group of adults, then on a small group of children, and finally on a larger group of 3,000 children. The researchers were pleased that in all these tests, the levels of antibodies in the blood went up, and that no ill effects were observed among the children. The two researchers declared that 'formalin inactivated virus is probably a perfectly safe vaccine...' The numbers of children used in the test were however far too small to make such a definitive judgement. The methods used to create the vaccine were far too risky to test on humans. Other researchers along with the scientific and medical establishment were horrified by what they saw as an ill-conceived and over hasty experiment. Many felt that Brodie and Park had rushed because they wanted to produce results before John Kolmer, who was also working on a vaccine in Philadelphia did. 'The race was on between Brodie and Kolmer as to which of their respective vaccines was to prove superior. Competition in this matter should not have been a factor which played a vital role; nevertheless it usually is, and certainly was in this particular instance,' John Paul, the Yale University polio researcher observed.[1]

Kolmer adopted a different, but perhaps riskier, approach and used a live but weakened form of the poliovirus for his vaccine, rather than a completely killed one. The scientific consensus then (and even now) is that infection with a live virus vaccine provides more lasting immunity than injection with a killed version of the virus. The challenge was to create a laboratory version of the virus that could not cause disease but would still be recognised by the immune system as a poliovirus. This would lead it to create antibodies that would protect against future infections from the real poliovirus. Kolmer's method of producing a weakened version of the virus was to take the spinal cord of monkeys infected with polio (which would contain poliovirus), grind and purify this material, treat it with a variety of chemicals including glycerol, sodium ricinoleate and phenyl mercury nitrate and store the mixture in a refrigerator at 12 to 16 degrees centigrade for ten to fourteen days. This process, he believed, destroyed the poliovirus' ability to cause paralytic disease, but left the virus potent enough to stimulate the immune system. Critics described Kolmer's hastily prepared vaccine, as a witches' brew. But he was able to persuade public health authorities in the United States and Canada to allow him to test the vaccine on 10,000 children.[2]

Kolmer's test created even more of a backlash in the scientific community than Park's and Brodie's because of fairly strong evidence that his vaccine had actually caused polio in children. He tested the vaccine in places where there were no outbreaks of polio at the time, but twelve children who were given his vaccine developed paralysis, and six of them died. It was possible that some of these cases might have contracted the disease naturally, but it appeared more probable that the vaccine had caused the disease. As a US Public Health Service official described it, 'Paralytic poliomyelitis was not epidemic at any of the localities at the time of occurrence of any of these cases....the likelihood of whole series of cases having occurred through these natural causes is extremely small. Although any of these cases may have been entirely unconnected with the vaccine the implication of the series as a whole is clear.'[3]

The way both groups of researchers had jumped from animal tests to tests on humans was thought to be overhasty. Evidence that one of the vaccines had caused paralysis in a small number of recipients brought the wrath of the scientific establishment down on the vaccine creators. At a convention in 1935, James Leake of the US Public Health Service accused Kolmer of committing murder.[4] The backlash against these hasty attempts to create a vaccine made scientists reluctant to continue. John Paul of Yale University, who was a prominent member of the polio research community at the time wrote, 'The events of 1935 cut more deeply into progress in the immunisation of man against poliomyelitis than most people realized at the time. It put an immediate stop to human vaccine trials that was to last for more than fifteen years—so dramatically and traumatically had the research programs of a whole generation of researchers on the immunisation problem been jolted.'[5]

Both groups of researchers had clearly been hasty and sloppy. Paul reflects the scientific consensus at the time when he writes, 'The crude non-quantitative methods used in virus inactivation might be described as "kitchen chemistry".' He describes the use of monkey spinal cord as 'far from ideal as it could cause encephalitis.'[6] The researchers also ignored evidence that the poliovirus had more than one serotype, and a vaccine that protected against one serotype would not be effective against other serotypes.

Yet the shock that the medical establishment expressed at these early experiments was in its own way perhaps slightly overblown. Decades later, the Salk and Sabin vaccines, though based on far more careful and painstaking scientific work, were also not incident free. When the Salk vaccine first went into production, one of the manufacturers, Cutter

Laboratories, had produced batches of vaccine where the poliovirus had not been fully inactivated, leading to children developing polio. Similarly, the Sabin vaccine caused occasional cases.

Despite the horror they evoked, the techniques used in the Park-Brodie and the Kolmer vaccines foreshadowed the work of Jonas Salk and Albert Sabin. Salk followed the route that Park-Brodie had taken and worked on a killed virus vaccine, while Sabin, like Kolmer worked on a live virus vaccine. The vital difference was that in the 1950s Salk and Sabin (perhaps because of the experience of the ill-fated earlier vaccines) were infinitely more careful. Perhaps equally crucially they benefited from knowledge about the poliovirus that was not available in the 1930s.

* * *

Jonas Salk was always a bit of an outsider among the prominent medical researchers of the time. As a son of Jewish immigrants from Tsarist Russia, Salk was never fully part of the Ivy-League-educated elite that dominated medical science (as well as almost every other facet of American life) in the early part of the last century. The top medical schools had tacit quotas restricting admission of Jewish students, and Salk had qualified from Bellevue Hospital Medical College in New York. This was a respectable school, but still considered a cut below the Ivy League medical schools at Harvard, Yale and Columbia. He was a hard-working and talented researcher whose work on an influenza vaccine during the Second World War had attracted attention. But as one of his biographers observes, he had still not been fully accepted into the inner circle of top rate virologists.[7]

Salk had cut his teeth as a researcher under Thomas 'Tommy' Francis Jr, one of the pioneers in the study of the influenza virus. The 1918 influenza pandemic had taken a huge toll on US soldiers during the First World War, and after the US entered the Second World War, one of the military's priorities was to protect its troops from flu attacks. Francis was made director of the US military's Commission on Influenza and charged with, among other things, developing an influenza vaccine. Salk joined Francis' laboratory at the University of Michigan, where he learned the tools and techniques that he would later use in creating a polio vaccine.

THE SALK VACCINE

In theory, a vaccine is easy to make. The virus (or bacteria) that causes a disease first needs to be cultivated in a lab. Then it needs to be either killed, or weakened in some way so that it does not cause disease. After that it needs to be tested first in animals, and then in humans for safety and finally for efficacy (or how effectively it would protect against the disease).

In practice, each of these steps is complex and prone to failure. A reliable method first needs to be found to grow large quantities of virus in the laboratory. The influenza virus was grown in chicken eggs. Salk learned to grow it in the lab by injecting eggs with small amounts of virus and incubating them for two days. At the end of this period he would lift off the top of the eggs and draw out the embryonic fluid which by then would be rich in newly multiplied flu virus. Then the virus had to be separated from the rest of the embryonic fluid and purified. The influenza vaccine that the Francis lab developed was a killed virus vaccine, so the next stage saw the virus from the embryo being killed by being dunked in formaldehyde. This killed virus mixed in a water or oil-based solution, was the vaccine.

Influenza, like polio, had more than one strain that infected humans, and so vaccines had to be created for different strains. Salk learned to test the safety of the vaccines as well as their effectiveness in preventing disease, first in small trials in humans to test safety, and then in larger trials to test efficacy. Salk was working for the military, and so trials were conducted on soldiers, who were in many ways ideal subjects, since they obeyed orders, turned up on time for vaccination and were always available for follow-up studies. Soldiers who had received the vaccine were compared with those who had not to see how much protection the vaccine offered. Inoculated soldiers were also tested over several years, to see how long the antibodies created by the vaccine persisted in the blood, and at what intervals booster shots might be necessary to increase diminishing antibody levels.

Each of these processes was long and laborious and Salk was to spend the best part of a decade working with Francis on influenza vaccines. This was ideal preparation for the work that was to catapult Salk to worldwide acclaim as the creator of the first effective vaccine against polio. John Paul writes that the period Salk spent working on influenza made him an expert in the technicalities of vaccine production as well as methods to evaluate the efficacy of vaccines. 'This experience alone would have been more than enough to qualify him as an ideal person to pursue a similar program to test a vaccine against poliomyelitis.'[8]

Salk's coming of age as a researcher and vaccine creator coincided with a series of polio epidemics in the immediate post war years when a vaccine against polio had become a priority for the NFIP. The leading polio scientists, perhaps still traumatised by the fallout from the Park-Brodie and Kolmer vaccine trials more than a decade earlier, were hesitant to risk their reputations in continuing the quest to develop a vaccine. In Jonas Salk, the NFIP and its head, Basil O'Connor, found a researcher who was not only willing to take the plunge, but also had the necessary experience.

Salk first came to attention in the world of polio research in 1948 when he took responsibility for a project that was an essential prerequisite for vaccine development. This involved determining how many different antigenic variants of the poliovirus existed in nature, since vaccines would have to be developed for each type. In 1931, the Australian researchers Frank Burnet and Jean Macnamara had found that there were at least two types of poliovirus that were antigenically distinct. So infection by one strain did not protect you from infection by another strain. But researchers in the United States paid little attention to this finding. Australia was considered a distant outpost of scientific learning. As one historical account of polio research commented, 'The report was treated with scepticism (in the United States) as it came from unknown investigators on a remote continent.'[9]

But by the 1950s, as pressure grew for a vaccine to be developed, it was clear that an essential first step was to discover how many types of poliovirus existed in nature. The work involved was laborious and mechanical, and the more well-known names in polio research, including Albert Sabin, were unwilling to get involved in what was seen as work that any competent laboratory technician could accomplish. But Salk was eager to plunge in, attracted by the funding from NFIP that would allow him to start his own laboratory at the University of Pittsburgh.

Poliovirus samples from all over the country poured into Salk's laboratory after the project began in November 1949. At the time two types of poliovirus were known to exist: Type 1 and Type 2. Salk's task was to determine whether any other types existed. To do this, monkeys were first injected with known Type 1 and Type 2 viruses. After a few days, their blood serum would contain antibodies to the type with which they had been injected. This serum was then collected. When any poliovirus of an unknown type arrived at Salk's laboratory in Pittsburgh, it would be mixed with Type 1 serum. The resultant mixture was injected into a monkey's brain (a procedure that involved pulling back the skin on the monkey's head, drilling a hole in its skull and then injecting in the virus and antibody mixture). If the monkey showed no signs of paralysis after this, it meant that the Type 1 antibody in the serum had killed the virus, which meant that the unknown virus was Type 1. If the monkey did become paralysed, it meant that the virus was not Type 1, since the Type 1 antibody had not neutralised the virus.

In this case, the virus would then be mixed with the Type 2 antibody, and injected into another monkey's brain. If the monkey survived this, then the unknown virus was Type 2. If it became paralysed, this meant the virus was neither Type 1 or 2, but a new type. By 1951, when the typing project ended, only one new type, dubbed Type 3, had been discovered through this process. It was therefore correctly concluded that the poliovirus only existed in three serotypes and that vaccines would have to be developed for all three types.

By then, a method to grow polioviruses in the laboratory had been discovered. Viruses, unlike bacteria, were hard to grow in artificial conditions. While bacteria did not need living cells in which to reproduce and would grow in a variety of nutritive media, viruses only reproduced in living cells. And they were also fussy about which kinds of cells in which they would replicate. Scientists had learned to grow cells as varied as embryonic chicken heart cells, monkey kidney cells and monkey testes cells in test tubes, but poliovirus would not grow in any of these.

Most laboratory work in the first half of the last century was done by growing poliovirus in monkeys and chimpanzees, killing the animals, and then harvesting their spinal cords or brains for the virus. This was an expensive and tedious process, and the right breeds of monkey—including the Indian rhesus and the cynomolgus—were not available to cultivate poliovirus on a scale that was large enough to create and test a vaccine.

In 1949, John Enders at Harvard University and his colleagues Thomas Weller and Fredrick Robbins were jointly awarded the Nobel

Prize for Medicine for devising a method to grow poliovirus easily. According to their method it was cultivated in a variety of human embryonic cell tissues in laboratory flasks filled with nutrient fluids that were changed every three to four days. The flasks were rotated gently at frequent intervals to ensure that the virus was evenly distributed over the cell medium.

Enders' discovery, along with his colleagues discovery, provided a much better way to grow large quantities of poliovirus in the laboratory, free of bacteria and other contaminants. As a result, all the techniques essential to creating a vaccine were in place.

The only remaining question was what kind of vaccine should be developed: a vaccine that used a killed, or inactivated, poliovirus, or a vaccine that used a weakened, or attenuated, form of the poliovirus? The consensus, from the time of Edward Jenner, the creator of the first smallpox vaccine, was that the most effective and long-lasting protection is provided by live virus vaccines. Indeed, the leading polio virologists of the time, including John Enders and Albert Sabin, all favoured a live virus vaccine. The successful vaccines produced during that period—such as the yellow fever vaccine, or the smallpox vaccine—were based on live viruses. Killed vaccines were thought to be less effective and more dangerous than live virus vaccines because it was felt there was no guarantee that live viral particles would not remain in the vaccine.

However, Salk's experience with influenza vaccines during the Second World War had convinced him that killed virus vaccines could be safely produced, and that with booster shots, these vaccines could provide lifelong immunity from the disease. He also flipped the argument about vaccine safety by pointing out that using a live vaccine version of the poliovirus could also be dangerous. What guarantee would there be that the mutations that had been introduced in the lab to weaken the virus would be effective, or that the virus would not revert to a disease-causing state?

Assisted by a talented team of junior researchers including Julius Youngner, who would go onto become a prominent virologist in his own right, Salk established a production facility for poliovirus in his laboratory at Pittsburgh. This was based on a modified version of Enders' tissue culture technique using monkey kidney cells. John

Troan, a Pittsburgh-based journalist who had access to Salk's laboratory described the virus making process: a monkey from Salk's laboratory (either a rhesus from India or a cynomolgous from the Philippines) would be anaesthetised, and its kidneys removed. The kidneys would then be chopped up into tiny fragments, rinsed in a salt solution to remove any remaining blood then suspended in the enzyme trypsin, to separate out individual cells. After that the liquid was kept at body temperature for ten minutes before being poured into a blender that would churn it until kidney cells rose to the top. The cells were then centrifuged, bathed in a nutrient solution and placed in glass flasks where they would grow for a week or so. Following this they were seeded with poliovirus, placed in incubators and gently rocked to ensure that the virus was evenly distributed. Within days, the virus would grow in the kidney cells, and eventually destroy them until a clear liquid brimming with poliovirus—pure naked virus, as Salk described it, would be left behind.[10]

Salk needed to experiment to solve two issues. One was to ensure that every last viral particle was completely killed by formalin, but in such a way that the structure of the virus would still be recognisable by the immune system as poliovirus. The other issue was to decide which strains of virus should be included in the vaccine. Vaccines would be created for all three strains of poliovirus, but there were variations within each strain, with some more virulent than others. Thanks to his involvement in the poliovirus typing project, Salk had a wide range of poliovirus to choose from. He needed to decide which strains would result in the most effective vaccine.

Salk's description of how he killed the virus provides a glimpse of how complex even something that apparently simple can be. The goal was to ensure that in any given lot of inactivated virus, not a single infectious particle remained. The four variables that needed to be controlled were the concentration of formaldehyde in the solution, the temperature at which the reaction was to take place, the pH, or acidity of the mixture, and the amount of virus that needed to be inactivated.[11]

The smallest of factors could alter the chances of inactivation. If there were still tiny particles of tissue from the laboratory culture in the viral mixture, this could shield the virus from the formaldehyde. Similarly, any bacteria or mould that had slipped into the tissue culture could also reduce the effectiveness of the inactivation, as well as introduce contaminants into the vaccine. Virus from tissue culture had to be filtered twice, including through bacteria-retaining filter pads. Since pH, or acidity was important for inactivation, either hydrochloric acid or acetic acid was added to the solution to bring it to the right levels. As the quantities of virus in each batch differed, a small portion would be removed and tested with formalin to determine how much time would be required to inactivate it.

Once this was determined, the batch would be treated with formalin for longer than the time deemed necessary to kill all the virus, to ensure that there was absolutely no chance of any live virus remaining. 'In order to destroy all the virus, so that some might not be missed by a chance selection of a sample for safety test, the reaction is allowed to proceed beyond the additional time required to destroy all infectious virus in the volume of material being tested,' Salk wrote.[12] Finally, each inactivated batch would be tested through injection into monkeys' brains. The monkeys would be watched for twenty-eight days, and if they did not develop paralysis, it was concluded that the batch of vaccine contained no live virus.

It was of course not enough that the vaccine was safe. It also had to be effective and produce a vigorous antibody response in the blood. Vaccine strains were injected into monkeys, and the level of antibody in their blood was measured. The strains were also injected into chimps, one step closer on the evolutionary ladder to humans to test the response.

By the early 1950s, Salk had vaccine strains that seemed safe and effective in monkeys and in chimps. The logical next step was to test it on human subjects. The primary concern in moving from animal to human tests, is to ensure that that vaccine does not cause harm. Salk's first trial was among a group of children living in a home for crippled children who had already had a bout of polio. Because of this the risk of them contracting polio from the vaccine was greatly reduced.

Salk chose fifty-two children whose parents had consented to their participation in the trial. He injected each one himself, and was relieved to find that none of them had any ill effects except redness at the injection site.[13] They were then given a second booster shot six weeks later, and their antibody levels were tested. The children all had increased antibody responses to the three types of poliovirus.

Salk then proceeded to another small-scale test at an institution for mentally disabled children, the Polk School, outside Pittsburgh. From Salk's point of view, there were advantages to testing the vaccine on institutionalised children. The children lived in a secluded, controlled environment, they had complete medical records, and they could be relied upon to be always present for routine blood tests and vaccinations. Also, since they rarely left the institution, many of the children had never been exposed to polio and were free of any antibodies to the virus. This made them ideal subjects to test the immunising effect of his vaccine.

The ethics of clinical testing were laxer in the 1950s than today, but there was still unease in the NFIP and the Pennsylvania state authorities about giving permission for experiments on children who were unable to provide informed consent. On top of this, in many cases they had no parents or guardians who could give such consent on their behalf. As Tom Rivers, one of the leading medical scientists of the time put it, 'An adult can do what he wants, but the same does not hold true for a mentally defective child. Many of these children did not have any mommas and poppas, or if they did their mommas and papas didn't give a damn about them.'[14] Salk found an ally however in the head of the Polk School, Gale Walker, who made a case to his superiors in the state government that the vaccine could be seen as a safety measure that would protect the children from polio.'[15]

Salk received permission and tested a variety of different approaches to vaccination. Some children received a vaccine with a mineral adjuvant [a substance that enhances the body's immune response], and others with the vaccine in an aqueous solution. Some were injected with a vaccine against single serotype, while others received a vaccine with all three serotypes. Salk was encouraged by the results: no one suffered any side effects beyond soreness at the site of the injection, and all reported encouraging levels of antibody response to polio.

These tests were an important proof of the concept that a vaccine using an inactivated vaccine could produce levels of antibody that in theory would be high enough to protect against polio. As Salk reported in a paper published in the *American Journal of Public Health* in 1954, his tests had shown that his vaccine provided antibody levels that were in many instances close to the antibody levels of those who had a natural polio infection. Since anyone who had been infected by polio once was protected from subsequent infections, it could be inferred that a vaccine that produced antibody levels similar to a natural infection, would also be protective. Salk also demonstrated that antibodies from vaccination persisted at least up to seven months. Equally significantly, a later booster shot resulted in a sharp rise in antibody levels. The crucial question that needed still to be determined was whether the antibody that the vaccine produced was sufficient to protect in real world conditions. Or, as Salk put it, the question to be determined was whether 'a procedure that induces antibody of a certain level [can] have a corresponding effect in the prevention of the paralytic disease.'[16] Only a large-scale test, under real world conditions, where children would be exposed to natural outbreaks of polio, would tell how effective the vaccine was.

In 1955, in what would be described as the largest public health experiment in American history, almost 1.5 million children participated in the clinical trial of Jonas Salk's vaccine. The NFIP chose Thomas Francis Jr, Salk's old mentor and a man known for his scientific integrity, to independently design and carry out the trials.

The trials were conducted using two separate methods. One would be a randomised controlled trial in which some children would receive the Salk vaccine, while others would receive an injected placebo. The choice of who would receive the vaccine and who would receive a placebo would be statistically randomised. Neither the child, nor the person administering the vaccine would know whether a placebo or the real vaccine was being given. This kind of randomised, blinded trial, is regarded as the gold standard of clinical trials. It eliminates biases—conscious and unconscious among researchers and trial administrators—on who should and should not get the vaccine. It also made it easier to control for social and economic variables such as gender, class and race.

But randomised trials can also pose an ethical dilemma. At a point when polio epidemics were rampant, would it be right to withhold a potentially life-saving injection from a child, and give the child a placebo instead? Salk argued that it would be unethical. He suggested an observational trial in which all children in a particular age group would be given the vaccine. Then the number of cases of polio in this group could be observed and compared to those among groups of children in other age groups who did not receive the vaccine. This meant that both types of trial were used. In some parts of the country, school children in the second grade (seven-year-olds in their second year of school) were given the vaccine, while children in the first and third grade were not given any vaccine and used as controls. In other parts of the country, first, second and third graders were injected with either polio vaccine or with placebo. The trials were scheduled for the polio low season in 1954, between March and June, so that the degree of protection that the vaccine offered could be measured during the summer months, when polio outbreaks were common.

The scientific basis for the trial was straightforward and followed traditional protocols for observational and experimental clinical trials. But the scale of the trial, as well as the operational and logistical challenges, were unprecedented. School districts, school heads, teachers and parents had to be contacted and brought on board. Communication material as well as consent forms had to be carefully put together in a way that would convince people to participate, without covering up any of the potential risks involved. Then there were the logistics of getting three doses of vaccine or placebo into roughly 650,000 school children. This involved keeping track of who had received the vaccine and who had received the placebo, making sure that the blood samples were collected and sending them to the right laboratory for analysis. Ensuring this was all tabulated properly was complex, with little margin for error.

Even producing vaccine for the trial was not easy. Since Salk's laboratory did not have enough capacity, two pharmaceutical companies—Eli Lily and Parke Davis—were licensed to produce the vaccine. Potential hitches quickly became clear. Salk discovered that the companies did not always follow his meticulous instructions, and the vaccine produced by both companies was producing polio when injected into monkeys. Salk visited both production facilities. At Parke Davis he found that they had shortened the time the live poliovirus had been exposed to formalin, and as a result not all the viral particles had been inactivated. At Eli Lily meanwhile, the virus had not been filtered properly before being placed in formalin, leaving particles of tissue and debris that interfered with the inactivation.[17]

As John Paul wrote, 'probably never in the history of medicine has a new public health measure been tested on such a wide scale, and so thoroughly. There were many risks involved in vaccinating so many, but as events turned out the trial succeeded. It was worth the tremendous effort involved.'[18]

It took nearly a year after the trials began for all the results to be tabulated and the statistical analysis completed. More than a hundred statisticians, coding experts and tabulating machine operators were involved. Working in the era before large scale computing and software were in use, they needed to enter and calculate around 144 million bits of information. Thomas Francis Jr, who was running the trial, insisted on strict secrecy until he was ready to release the results. Neither Salk, nor the NFIP, nor the public had any inkling of what they would be. Finally, on 12 April 1955, a date that fell on the tenth anniversary of Franklin Roosevelt's death, Francis announced the results at a widely anticipated conference at the University of Michigan. The Salk vaccine was safe, and effective, and ready to use. He delivered a one-and-a-half-hour-long presentation, delivered in a dry academic monotone, replete with charts and slides.

The most crucial data on vaccine effectiveness came about an hour into his presentation. Among the 749,000 children in the placebo controlled study, thirty-three children from the vaccinated group had developed polio, compared to 110 in the placebo group. This meant that the rate of polio among the unvaccinated was approximately 3.3 times greater than in the vaccinated. Overall, the vaccine was 80–90 per cent effective against paralytic poliomyelitis, with some variation among the vaccine strains. The Type 1 vaccine was only 60–70 per cent effective, while the Type 2 and Type 3 was 90 per cent effective. In summation, Francis declared, 'Properly prepared vaccine of the Salk variety is safe, antigenically potent and has a high degree of effectiveness in the prevention of paralytic poliomyelitis.[19]

Newspaper headlines the next day reflected the immensity of the achievement. 'Polio Conquered', declared the *Pittsburgh Press*, in a headline that typified the media reaction. *The New York Times* devoted several pages of its 13 April 1955 edition to the announcement and its impact, and declared in its editorial that this development was 'a turning point in medical history…Gone are the old helplessness, the fear of an invisible enemy, the frustration of physicians. Gone too are the hot-weather epidemics of poliomyelitis. Science has enriched mankind with one of its finest gifts.'

THE SALK VACCINE

Jonas Salk instantly became a national hero. As *Time* magazine wrote in his obituary in 1995, finding a vaccine against polio turned him into one of the most celebrated men of the 1950s. Contemporary opinion polls ranked him with Gandhi and Churchill as one of the most celebrated men of the time.

Six companies were licensed to produce the vaccine, and within weeks, mass immunisation campaigns were held in schools and other locations, the process only held up by the inability of the manufacturers to produce enough vaccine. A tragic blip occurred when one of the laboratories producing vaccine, Cutter laboratory in California, let improperly inactivated vaccine onto the market, paralysing over 204 children. Safety procedures and inspections of vaccine manufacturing facilities were tightened, and the Salk vaccine soon established itself as one of the safest vaccines in use. It ended the terror of polio in the United States and everywhere else it was used as the number of cases of polio dropped dramatically. In 1954, the year before the Salk vaccine was introduced, there were over 38,000 cases of polio reported. By 1961 this had come down to a little over a 1,000 cases.

* * *

The Salk vaccine transformed polio in the United States and Western Europe from one of the biggest threats to child health, to a preventable childhood disease, like measles or mumps. But it was not considered a tool to eradicate polio by exterminating the poliovirus. The vaccine did not prevent infection by the poliovirus; it only prevented paralysis. This was because someone protected by the vaccine could still get infected by the poliovirus, but the vaccine would then create antibodies that stopped the virus from entering the blood stream and attacking the nerves of the spinal cord. The vaccine turned the poliovirus from a potential paralyser, to another harmless enteric virus that replicated briefly in humans without causing harm, before exiting the human body either through the faeces or through respiratory droplets to infect fresh human hosts. The Salk vaccine was an excellent tool to protect children from polio. But because it did not prevent the virus from replicating in humans, it was not seen as a tool for eradication or a permanent solution to the problem of polio.

Salk himself disputed this view, and maintained that with high rates of vaccination, the poliovirus would eventually be exterminated and eradication would be achieved. But this was not the prevailing opinion among epidemiologists. Had the Salk vaccine been the only one developed in the United States, it is unlikely a global eradication campaign would have been embarked upon by the WHO. It required another, unique, vaccine to open the possibility of worldwide elimination.

4

A TOOL FOR ERADICATION

ALBERT SABIN AND THE ORAL POLIO VACCINE

It was early on a January morning in 1955, barely hours after an over-night storm had coated the highways in ice and blanketed the country-side in snow. Albert Sabin took his life in his hands and drove over a hundred miles across the treacherous roads from his home in Cincinnati to a penitentiary for young offenders in the town of Chillicothe. Sabin could have waited a day or two when conditions would have been bet-ter and the journey less risky. But this would have gone entirely against his character. Sabin was a driven, ambitious man, and was not going to allow a snowstorm to stand between him and the goal on which he had set his sights. That goal was to develop a revolutionary new polio vac-cine that would eliminate the disease for all time. To achieve this, his most immediate task was to get to the penitentiary, come what may, and ask for permission to test his vaccine on the inmates.

Sabin, aged 49, was already one of the foremost medical researchers of his time, with a list of accomplishments that would have taken others a lifetime to achieve. As an army doctor during the Second World War, he had developed vaccines for strains of encephalitis and dengue, two diseases that affected US soldiers in the tropics. In the post-war years he had established himself as a leading polio researcher, with a well-funded research programme and a prestigious position at the University of Cincinnati's Children's Hospital.

51

But Sabin was also deeply frustrated. His mission to develop a polio vaccine using a live, weakened form of the poliovirus was receiving little encouragement from the public or from the powerful National Foundation for Infantile Paralysis (NFIP), the chief funder and arbiter of all work on polio in the United States. His rival Jonas Salk's vaccine on the other hand, had just been tested on over a million American children, in the largest clinical trial the world had seen. Data from the trial was still being evaluated, but all the buzz was around the Salk vaccine which was seen as the magic bullet that would end the epidemics of polio that swept the United States every summer.

Sabin neither approved of Salk's vaccine, nor of Jonas Salk himself, whom he considered to be a second-rate researcher. The Salk vaccine used poliovirus that had been killed, or inactivated and Sabin had several objections to a killed virus vaccine. Like many other scientists, Sabin was convinced that the immunity conferred by a killed virus vaccine would be temporary, and repeated booster shots would be required to confer longterm protection from the disease. He felt that only a vaccine based on a live virus would confer lifelong immunity. Besides being ineffective, Sabin also thought that Salk's vaccine was potentially dangerous because it included a particularly virulent strain of Type 1 poliovirus. He argued that there was no guarantee that a few live particles might remain in the vaccine.

Never one to keep his disagreements private or avoid a confrontation, Sabin had publicly expressed his misgivings about the Salk vaccine on several occasions. Shortly after 5,000 children in Pittsburgh had received the Salk vaccine as part of a clinical trial, Sabin criticised the vaccine in an interview to the *New York Times*. He declared that the trials were being conducted in haste, and that the Salk vaccine might not be safe. He also adroitly used the interview to tout the benefits of the live virus vaccine that he was working on. His vaccine, unlike Sabin's would produce immunity for a long time, perhaps even lifelong immunity, he said.[1]

Sabin's quest was also no doubt spurred by competitiveness. He knew that Hilary Koprowski—another well-known polio researcher at the pharmaceutical company Lederle—had, five years earlier tested a live virus vaccine at a home for mentally disabled children at Letchworth in New York State. For a while, it was a toss-up as to whether Koprowski or Sabin would produce the more widely accepted vaccine. Sabin won out in the end, but the race was close.

Koprowski, like Sabin was a brilliant but temperamental individual and an undercurrent of rivalry flowed between these two Polish-born Jewish immigrants to the United States. Koprowski was a decade younger, but had produced a live vaccine poliovirus before Sabin had. After growing a weakened form of the poliovirus in mouse brains he had tested it on himself in 1948 and later at the home for mentally disabled children in 1950. The test results were encouraging: seventeen of the twenty children to whom the vaccine was administered developed antibodies to polio, and none of them developed any complications. Koprowski had shown that it was possible to produce an attenuated form of the poliovirus in the lab that, at least in preliminary tests, seemed safe enough to administer to humans.

News of Koprowski's tests were received with horror rather than hailed as a scientific breakthrough by others working on a polio vaccine, partly because testing a vaccine based on a live poliovirus was considered far too dangerous. A killed virus vaccine of the kind that Jonas Salk was developing and testing extensively on monkeys and chimpanzees seemed the way to go. Playing around with a vaccine based on a live virus that caused epidemics of paralysis was thought to be both risky and unnecessary when extensive work was going ahead on Salk's alternative. Koprowski had also tested the vaccine on mentally handicapped children with little or no capacity for informed consent, pushing against ethical boundaries.[2]

When he presented his findings to the big names in the world of polio research at a meeting organised by the NFIP, his results were received with silence. Most participants did not seem to know what to make of this attempt to use live poliovirus in a vaccine, without receiving any form of ethical approval. But Albert Sabin, who was present, was incensed by the risks that had been taken. He sought out Koprowski afterwards and chastised him, 'How dare you feed live poliovirus to children.'[3]

Koprowski was undaunted. If a vaccine was to be developed, it had to be tested somewhere, and someone had to take the first step towards testing. Later he would admit that he could have gone to jail for those tests and the company could have been sued. But he justified his actions on the basis that that the history of medicine and vaccine development were filled with similar tests on institutionalised children. Koprowski had followed his initial tests by continuing to develop and refine his viral strains, and his vaccine was eventually tested in large-scale human trials in the then Belgian colonies of Congo, Rwanda and Burundi.

Despite Sabin's angry confrontation with Koprowski, the two maintained cordial relations, exchanging samples, visiting each other's labs, and even inviting each other to their homes, as Koprowski did when Sabin visited the Lederle lab in 1953. But underneath these courteous exchanges, the rivalry between these two strong personalities ran deep. Neither man wanted to lose to the other in the unspoken competition to produce the safest and most effective live virus vaccine.

Sabin's own vaccine would be put to largescale use in the Soviet Union. Around the same time Koprowski maintained that he had provided the viral samples that Sabin used to develop some of his vaccine strains, wryly describing himself as the founder of the Sabin vaccine. Sabin was influenced and perhaps secretly impressed by Koprowski's development of an oral vaccine nearly a decade ahead of his own efforts. But in public he could be dismissive of Koprowski, contrasting his own, painstaking work with what he claimed were his rival's more slapdash efforts.

Koprowski resented these slights on his scientific ability, and the relationship between the two broke down in 1958. This was after Sabin tested Koprowski's vaccine samples in his lab on monkeys and declared they were far more virulent than Koprowski had reported. In a veiled barb, Sabin wondered whether Koprowski's lab assistant had incorrectly reported the results.[4] The incensed Koprowski, shot back a letter stating that three laboratories had independently corroborated his vaccine's safety, and that he found Sabin's letter most extraordinary. Koprowski, who was extremely well read, began his letter by quoting the fifteenth century Dutch theologian Thomas a Kempis, implying that it was Sabin's ego and vanity that were causing him to question the safety of the Koprowski vaccine. 'If you aspire to reach this height of perfection, you must make a brave beginning. Lay the axe to the roots, to cut out and destroy all inordinate and secret love of self, and of any personal and material advantage. From the vice of inordinate self-love spring nearly all those other failings that have to be completely overcome,' he advised.[5] An incandescent Sabin, not to be outdone in the literary quotation department, shot back a curt letter with a brief line from Shakespeare, 'The devil can quote Scriptures...' declaring, 'You impugn my motives, veracity and honour. Farewell my one time friend and colleague.'[6]

Science tends to be seen as a dispassionate quest for an objective reality, conducted by rational human beings impervious to the emotions, ambitions and egocentric biases that afflict other people. But as should be obvious, scientists are cut from the same cloth as the rest of human society and riven by the same human frailties and failings. The scientific method, is commonly understood as a cycle of observation, hypothesis and experiment. But it is human beings, not machines, who carry out this cycle of knowledge acquisition. Experiments are conducted by human hands, some superbly skilled, others less so, and the results are measured and interpreted by minds often clouded by human foible. Despite this, science has provided for us a map of the workings of the natural world that is reliable enough to build bridges and roads, develop drugs and vaccines and send satellites to the farthest reaches of the solar system.

But the explanatory power of science runs dry when it runs into the shifting sands of human decision making. It does not tell us for example why at the end of the day, Sabin's vaccine rather than Koprowski's vaccine became widely used globally. Both vaccines had been tested extensively on humans without ill effect. Joseph Melnick, a respected virologist at Baylor University in Texas, tested Koprowski's and Sabin's as well as a third set of live vaccine strains produced by Herald Cox, an erstwhile collaborator of Koprowski. He found all the samples he tested to be more virulent when injected into the spinal cords and brains of monkey's than the vaccines' developers had stated. Sabin's, Koprowski's and Cox's vaccine viruses all produced some degree of illness after these injections.

Virulence in monkeys is not the same as virulence in human beings (as both Sabin and Koprowski were fond of pointing out), but this was the only yardstick that could be used at the time to measure the safety of the vaccine virus. Sabin's strains were slightly less virulent to monkeys than Koprowski's strains, and therefore found favour with the US regulatory authorities and the WHO.

Had the Koprowski vaccine found favour for widespread use, it might well have caused fewer side effects in humans and been more efficient in eradicating polio in tropical countries than the Sabin vaccine. Both Koprowski's biographer, Richard Vaughan, and the historian of polio in America, David Oshinsky have suggested that Koprowski's role as an outsider working in private industry could have played a role in his vaccine falling by the wayside. Had Koprowski been a university based researcher rather than a researcher at a pharmaceutical company, the virology community might have received his work more favourably.[7] After Sabin's vaccine found favour in the United States and the WHO in the 1960s, Koprowski moved to other fields, including developing an improved rabies vaccine, and developing the use of monoclonal antibodies in disease treatment. He was in many ways the pioneer of the live virus vaccine, the tool that would eventually be used for global eradication. But it was Sabin's vaccine that was eventually used, and it is Sabin's work that we need to follow to understand the quest to eradicate polio.

* * *

Albert Sabin always maintained that his approach towards creating a safe poliovirus vaccine was more meticulous and painstaking than Koprowski's, or for that matter anyone else working on poliovirus at the time. He attributed this in part to his early experience as a researcher at the Rockefeller Institute in New York, at a time when the ill-fated Park-Brodie and Kolmer vaccines were rushed into human tests without adequate studies on their safety. Part of Sabin's belief that the Salk vaccine was potentially unsafe, could be due to this early experience with killed virus vaccines.

The inspiration for Sabin's search for a live virus vaccine was the South African born Max Theiler, who won a Nobel Prize for developing a yellow fever vaccine based on a live, weakened, yellow fever virus.

Theiler's big discovery was that the characteristics of a virus could be changed by growing it in different animal tissues. If yellow fever virus was grown in mouse brain tissue for several generations, it developed new characteristics becoming more and more virulent for mice, but less and less virulent in monkeys, producing increasingly mild yellow fever symptoms. By growing yellow fever virus strains in different permutations and combinations of animal cells, primarily chick and mouse embryos, Theiler developed a virus strain that met the two criteria he was looking for. These were a loss of virulence in the visceral organs that were attacked by yellow fever in humans and monkeys, and a loss of ability to cause damage to the nervous system.

Theiler painstakingly selected strains by cultivating the virus in different animal tissue until he arrived at a vaccine virus that would be safe for humans. This provided the template for Koprowski and Sabin's work. Sabin would be one of those who would go on to nominate Theiler for the Nobel Prize, an acknowledgment perhaps of the influence he had on his thinking and work.

During the course of his work at the Rockefeller Institute, Theiler had already produced a strain of the poliovirus that had lost its virulence in monkeys after repeated passage in mice brains. Sabin had built on this to understand how the characteristics of a poliovirus changed with the kind of tissue in which it was cultivated.

The road to understanding these strains was a long, exhausting process. Today, molecular techniques allow researchers to alter a virus' characteristics by cutting or making additions to its genome. But in the pre-molecular era in which Theiler, Sabin and Koprowski worked, the only way to understand and alter a virus was through repeated cultivation in cell cultures and observing the changes that occurred. This involved cultivating hundreds of viral strains in the lab and injecting them into hundreds of monkeys, and killing and autopsying them to see what damage the virus had done.

Sabin used more monkeys and chimps in his labs than any of his contemporaries. and would run through a thousand monkeys in a year, repeatedly testing strains to ensure that the results were sound, and reproducible. In one year, 1952, he used 1,200 monkeys for his tests, and did all the post-mortem histological examinations himself. Other researchers, he said 'were accustomed to working with cultures in a laboratory, maybe a few monkeys, but with a few monkeys, you don't learn very much.'[8] Sabin on the other hand, who was always generously funded by the NFIP, had two floors of animal quarters in his lab at Cincinnati that could hold up to 350 monkeys, between twenty and forty chimpanzees, and thousands of mice.

Sabin was a hard taskmaster, but even his detractors acknowledged that he drove himself harder than he drove his research staff. Unlike other senior researchers who left matters like injecting monkeys and performing autopsies to their junior staff, Sabin did not delegate. 'He did all the work himself... he was extremely careful. He inoculated the monkeys in the same way, he sectioned them to look for lesions in the same way, he was just very meticulous,' recalls Vincent Racaniello, a professor of virology and a distinguished polio researcher.[9]

The twice-yearly reports that Sabin sent to his funder, the NFIP, meticulously details his experiments to create an ideal vaccine virus. A typical study involved testing the Mahoney strain, a particularly virulent strain of Type 1 poliovirus. Sabin began by administering it to twenty cynomolgus monkeys orally. Ninety per cent of them developed an infection, and sixty per cent of them were paralysed. He then took virus samples from the infected monkeys and grew them repeatedly in his laboratory in a culture of monkey kidney cells, harvesting each batch of virus and then regrowing it in fresh culture. Each batch of poliovirus had different characteristics: some, for example, would grow abundantly, others would grow more rapidly. Sabin tried to correlate these different characteristics to the virus's ability to cause paralysis and select viral strains that were least likely to cause paralysis. He discovered that the particles that reproduced the quickest in the lab seemed to have lost their capacity to produce paralysis in monkeys. From this, Sabin drew the lesson that rapid passaging in tissue could produce viral particles with reduced paralytic power in monkeys.[10]

From 1949 until 1955, when his oral vaccine was tested on a large scale outside the United States, Sabin and his associated conducted thousands of such experiments. These created different permutations and combinations of viruses and culturing methods to produce the kind of vaccine virus strains he was looking for. Such experiments gave Sabin an insight into the role evolution played in viral infections. He found that the further along the evolutionary tree of primates you went, the less lethal the poliovirus was to the nervous system, and the more it became an intestinal infection. Monkeys for example were very susceptible to paralytic disease when the virus was injected into their brains, but their intestines were resistant to the virus. Chimps, one evolutionary step closer to humans, were relatively more resistant than monkeys to the virus being injected in the brain, but more susceptible to intestinal infections than monkeys. Humans were the most susceptible to the virus as an intestinal infection, but far less susceptible than monkeys and chimps to developing paralytic polio.

This observation helped in identifying viral strains to use in a live vaccine. Since monkeys were more susceptible to paralysis than both chimps and humans, Sabin first identified strains that had very low paralytic effect when injected into the brains and spinal cords of monkeys. His lab received poliovirus samples from children all over the country, which he would then grow in monkey and human tissue. By rapidly passaging them through different cultures and then purifying the resulting strains, Sabin would separate out viral particles with different characteristics such as rapid growth, or strong pathogenic effects. Strains with the lowest levels of damage to monkey brain and spinal tissue would then be selected for testing on chimps, often after further growth in cell cultures.

Chimps would receive the vaccine orally, intramuscularly and injected directly into the anterior horn cells of their spinal cord. They would be observed for signs of paralysis, and blood would be drawn from them to see whether the virus had passed into the blood stream and antibodies were being produced. Their faeces would be tested to see how well different strains reproduced in their intestines. At the end of a fixed period, they would be killed and autopsied, and Sabin would look for lesions in the spinal cords that would indicate a poliovirus attack. The same experiments were often repeated several times over to ensure that the results were sound, and each result was meticulously noted. Sabin figured that a strain of the poliovirus that did not cause paralysis or lesions when injected straight into the spinal cord of a chimp, the primate closest to man, was unlikely to cause harm in humans. This could then provide the basis for a vaccine virus.

By the end of 1953, four years after he began his tests, Sabin had developed three types of weakened virus that produced no disease at all when injected into chimpanzees. He had also reached a stage where he could go no further without being able to test his vaccine viruses on humans. The big questions were whether these strains would multiply in human intestinal tracts and produce enough of an antibody response to protect against poliovirus infection. Only human trials could resolve these questions.

Sabin and two of his associates Dr Manuel Ramos Alvarez, a Mexican researcher and Hugh Harding a laboratory technician, tested the vaccine on themselves in early 1954. They each swallowed large doses of the vaccine virus, and waited to see what would happen. None of them suffered any ill effects, but blood and stool tests showed that the weakened viruses were doing what they were supposed to do. The virus reproduced in their intestines, and also provoked an antibody response in the blood. This gave Sabin the confidence he needed to propose larger trials to answer a variety of questions. Should the vaccine be given orally or injected intramuscularly? Would the different vaccine strains for the three serotypes interfere with each other if given together? What quantities of the vaccine virus would be excreted in the faeces? And would the excreted viruses remain benign, or would they re-acquire the ability to produce paralysis? He needed new human subjects to test to answer these questions, but this was proving to be difficult. With scientific and public attention focused on the Salk trials, the powers that be at the NFIP and its powerful head, Basil O Connor did not want to muddy the waters by testing another vaccine.

When he asked the NFIP for permission to begin human trials with three mild viral strains, the committee on Virus Research told him that it was 'not willing to recommend that you proceed with trials on human beings immediately.' Instead the NFIP's Director of Research, Henry Kumm had told Sabin that his proposal would go before the Vaccine Committee, but did not indicate when and whether the committee would meet. Kumm also urged 'the necessity of proceeding with great caution in situations such as this', and stressed the need to make arrangements for insurance should things go wrong.

Sabin argued, perhaps a little disingenuously, but fruitlessly, that he was not actually testing vaccines, but only trying to understand the behaviour of different weakened strains of poliovirus he had propagated in his laboratory. In the end, he was pragmatic enough to realise that he was unlikely to get permission in the year that the Salk vaccine was being tested, and said he would postpone his tests and reapply for permission at the end of 1954. As he later recalled in an oral history recorded by Saul Benison, 'In 1954, the NFIP was about as fully occupied as it could be at the so called Francis Field trials of Salk vaccine. The intrusion of any other kind of activity, of any other kind of vaccine was something they wished, like a bad dream might go away.'[11]

Sabin accepted that the powers that be were not in favour of trials for his vaccine, but he was also not one to let the grass grow under his feet. He began scouting for human subjects. He needed a place where he could get a sufficient number of volunteers for a sufficiently long period of time, who would be amenable to repeated drawing of blood and faeces, and who lived in a relatively closed, controlled environment. People who have been institutionalised or incarcerated tick all these boxes, which is why prisons, and care homes for juveniles and the mentally disabled figure so prominently in the history of medicine. While corresponding with the NFIP, Sabin had approached an institution for mentally disabled children in New York State, asking whether he could run experiments on the children, but was turned down.

Undaunted by his first rebuff, Sabin thought of using inmates at a penitentiary as volunteers for his study. The town of Chillicothe, close enough to Sabin's base in Cincinnati to allow him to supervise the study, had an institution for young offenders that seemed ideal. Sabin knew that a former associate of his, virologist Robert Huebner, was already doing studies in the institution on respiratory viruses, and so got in touch with James Bennett the director of federal prisons in Washington to ask for permission. The director, in turn asked Sabin to get approval from the medical director of the federal prison service, Dr H M Janney. Dr Janney then said Sabin would have to get approval from the warden of the penitentiary at Chillicothe, the ultimate arbiter of all that happened in the institution. Sabin wrote to the warden, a Dr Hagerman, who asked him to come to the penitentiary on a day early in the New Year, a day that happened to coincide with the snowstorm.

The conditions were treacherous, and Sabin was nervous about driving. 'I said to myself I am going to take my life in my own hands, because many of those were back roads, it wasn't main highway,' he recalled. 'And I said to myself that if I allow this snow storm and these icy roads to stop me at this moment, that will be very bad, because it may be only the beginning of many other points at which I may stop because of potential difficulties.'[12]

Sabin arrived late for his appointment. The drive in icy conditions took much longer than expected. But Sabin's determination paid off. The warden greeted him by saying that he had never expected him to come, and that he had already made up his mind to refuse permission for tests on the inmates. But he was impressed by Sabin making the trip under those conditions, and said he would give him a fair hearing. Sabin made his pitch to the warden, who told him 'I am going to give you permission to talk to the prisoners themselves. And if you can get volunteers from that tough bunch, all right.'[13]

Sabin stayed overnight at Chillicothe, and addressed the 2,000 odd prisoners the next morning. He was a scientist, accustomed to speaking to his peers in the language of science, but here he was speaking with a very different audience, 'a tough bunch' as the warden described them. Sabin recalled he told them the purpose of the experiments, and said they would be contributing to ending the scourge of polio forever. And as for any risks involved in the tests, he told them they would be far less than the risk to life and limbs that he had taken to drive to the penitentiary just after a snowstorm. He was convincing enough to persuade a long line of volunteers to sign up for the trials that would last for three years. The results would provide the scientific knowledge and experience that would eventually go into the vaccine that would be used to eradicate polio globally.

* * *

When he began in 1955, Sabin was not sure whether his vaccine should be given orally or injected, so both methods were tried in Chillicothe. But the antibody response was much lower when the viral strains were injected, and so the oral route was chosen, and the inmates were fed vaccine strains mixed in a sweet syrup. After receiving the vaccine the prisoners would be bled every few days to check the antibody response, and stool samples would be taken frequently to test that the vaccine virus was indeed reproducing in the intestine.

Blood and stool samples from Chillicothe would be tested in Sabin's lab in Cincinnati, and any viral samples with promising characteristics would be further passaged in tissue cultures, tested in monkeys and chimps, and perhaps retested on the prisoners. Sabin was also receiving virus samples from children with polio from across the United States, and was testing these for promising candidates for vaccine virus production.

By 1957, Sabin had completed most of his work at Chillicothe, and had developed three vaccine strains, one for each of the poliovirus serotypes, that he considered to be safe as well as immunogenic. It was now time to test these on larger populations living in open communities, including children. But before he did that, Sabin was duty bound to do one last test: on his two daughters, aged five and seven, along with three of their playmates and his wife Sylvia. Testing the vaccine on children, or adults for that matter, was not pleasant. The children needed to be bled at frequent intervals, and their stool samples needed to be collected regularly as well. 'What can you say to a five-year and seven-year-old, particularly when you have to stab them, and the needles were not that sharp in those days... and I had to bleed them before, bleed them at intervals... I said we are going to collect your faeces every day, or every other day. You are going to have to do it in a little container so I can take the stuff out. I'm going to have to bleed you... my poor children stood up very well because this was quite a period. ... it didn't mean they didn't cry, but by God when they went to the toilet, they did exactly as I wanted to do.'[14]

By now, Albert Sabin knew he was on the verge of developing a polio vaccine that had a significance larger than perhaps he himself had realised when he began his quest. He had created in the laboratory a live, weakened version of the poliovirus that mimicked the wild poliovirus in all but its capacity to cause paralysis. It induced in the human body the creation of antibodies that would protect against wild poliovirus. And since it was fed orally and mimicked the passage of the natural or wild poliovirus through the intestines, it also created an immune response in the human intestines. This meant that if someone who had been immunised by Sabin's vaccine virus was later infected with wild poliovirus, the virus would be attacked by the immune system in the intestine, and would not be able to reproduce. If it could not reproduce, the chain of transmission by which the poliovirus travelled from person to person causing disease would be broken.

This had revolutionary implications. A live virus vaccine that protected the intestine from future infection opened up the prospect of eradicating the natural poliovirus, and driving it to extinction. The poliovirus has only one home on earth: the human intestines. If enough intestines were protected across the world from poliovirus infection, the virus would be eradicated.

That potential for eradication was what distinguished Sabin vaccine from Jonas Salk's killed virus vaccine. The Salk vaccine protected individuals from disease, but did not stop them from being silent transmitters of the poliovirus. Sabin's vaccine virus, if disseminated widely across the world, could replace a naturally occurring virus, with an artificially created milder version. This was genetic engineering of the highest order: squeezing out a naturally occurring virus from its habitat by strains created in a laboratory. It was something that human beings had been doing for centuries when they bred plants and animals to evolve characteristics that they needed. Max Theiler's yellow fever vaccine virus had also been developed in the laboratory, but unlike the Sabin vaccine, it was injected into humans, and never left the human body. Sabin's vaccine would be let loose in the environment, to spread naturally the way wild poliovirus did.

It would be the first time that a virus had been bred in the laboratory that would spread naturally through the environment through the faecal oral route—just like the wild poliovirus but without causing paralysis.

But sending a lab-created vaccine virus into the wider environment created a huge challenge. These vaccine strains would always come out slightly altered by their passage through the human intestine. The fear was that they would re-acquire the ability to cause paralytic disease, and then infect others in the same way that wild poliovirus did. The challenge was to ensure that Sabin's strains were stable enough not to re-acquire neurovirulent characteristics, or cause disease themselves. 'It wouldn't do to create a new monster.' as he put it.[15]

While Sabin was convinced that he had created the ultimate weapon against polio, he found that his enthusiasm and excitement was not matched in the United States. No support was forthcoming either from the powers that be at the NFIP, or even others in the field of polio research. With the Salk vaccine coming into wide use in the United States, there was no real demand for a new vaccine. The NFIP felt that testing and introducing a new vaccine at that point in time was unnecessary, and would only confuse the public who had been told that the Salk vaccine was excellent. After the Cutter incident had temporarily destroyed public confidence in polio vaccines, the NFIP's sole focus at this point in time was to increase public confidence in the Salk vaccine, and encourage parents to vaccinate their children. Testing a new, and possibly controversial, vaccine was the last thing the Foundation wanted to get involved in. And without the NFIP's blessing, it was impossible to conduct large scale trials, particularly in the United States.

The cruellest blow came when Sabin's good friend and occasional collaborator, Tom Rivers, who was at the time medical director at the NFIP, told him bluntly to throw his vaccine down the drain and forget about it. As Sabin later put it, this rejection of his vaccine by a respected scientist and friend was traumatic.[16] Given the international role his vaccine would later have, it is only appropriate that it was interest from overseas that saved his vaccine from dying in obscurity in the United States.

* * *

In January 1956, while he was still busy with the trials at Chillicothe, Sabin had received a letter from a Dr H van Zile Hyde, at the US Department of Health, Education and Welfare. The letter told him about a proposed visit by a group of Soviet researchers to his laboratory at Cincinnati to see the work that he was doing on vaccines. The visit by the Soviet scientists was one sign of the small thaw in US-Soviet relations after the death of Stalin and during the Eisenhower administration. Official exchanges and visits between scientists were gradually resuming, with both governments also seeing this a good way to get intelligence on what the other side was doing.

Until a few years earlier, the Soviet Union, like most of the world outside the United States and Western Europe, had not experienced epidemics of polio, possibly because standards of hygiene were lower than in the West. As a consequence children were exposed to the virus early in life and received lifelong immunity. But in 1954, an epidemic swept the Soviet Union causing around 20,000 cases of paralysis. Two years later, another epidemic hit the country, and finding a way to control the disease became a priority. Jonas Salk's vaccine was being administered to the general public in the United States and the Soviets wanted to learn about the Salk vaccine so they could use it at home. But besides visiting Salk at Pittsburgh, they were also using their time in the United States to visit other polio researchers like Sabin.

The Soviet delegation comprised Mikhail Chumakov, Director of the Poliomyelitis Research Institute in Moscow and his wife and scientific collaborator Maria Konstantinova Voroshilova who worked with him at the Institute. They were accompanied by A A Smorodintsev, Director of the Department of Virology at the Institution of Experimental

Medicine at Leningrad. The meeting at Cincinnati went well and led to an invitation to Sabin to visit the USSR, which he accepted after getting permission from the US State Department.

This marked the beginning of a strong professional and personal relationship between Sabin and his Soviet visitors, in particular between Sabin and Chumakov. Later, when Sabin became a frequent visitor to the Soviet Union, he and Chumakov would have long arguments over the merits of communism and capitalism over bottles of vodka and caviar. Sabin would recall 'One glass of vodka and caviar, one after the other. Neither one giving into the other a fraction of an inch, ending up embracing and kissing each other in the Soviet fashion. That was the relationship.'[17]

The Soviets had decided earlier to produce the Salk vaccine, because of its track record in the United States, and Chumakov's institute in Moscow was turned into a testing and manufacturing centre for the vaccine. But the Russians also wanted to keep their options open, and Smorodintsev was asked to research the possibility of using live virus vaccines in Leningrad. Sabin provided seed supplies of the three attenuated vaccine strains, which Smorodintsev tested on children in Leningrad in 1957. The vaccine produced no side effects, and led to a strong antibody response. Since an oral vaccine was also much easier to administer to children than the Salk vaccine in 1959 large-scale use of Sabin's vaccine began in different parts of the Soviet Union. Between January and October that year, approximately 10 million children under the age of 15 received three doses of the Sabin vaccine, administered at monthly intervals.

Part of the trial period coincided with a polio outbreak in the Uzbek capital Tashkent and required the rapid use of the oral vaccine in a mass campaign. The strategy the Soviets used was a template for what would happen in other parts of the world once a global eradication campaign was launched. Several days before the campaign, announcements were made through local radio, television and newspapers to urge parents to keep their children at home to get vaccinated. On the day of the campaign, vaccination teams went house-to-house, giving two drops of vaccine containing all three serotypes to children under the age of 15. The vaccinations were carried out on three days in July and August. Six weeks after their first dose, a second dose was administered to children in the same way.

The Salk vaccine trials had been conducted under strict protocols to evaluate vaccine effectiveness by comparing those who had received the vaccine with control groups that had not received the vaccine. But the trials in the USSR were based on mass administration of the vaccine to all children. The Soviets took the view that at a time when polio epidemics were threatening children, it would not be right to withhold it from those in a control group and so everyone who was eligible received the vaccine.

Instead of a standard case control trial, Chumakov and his colleagues measured vaccine effectiveness by looking at the rise in antibody levels after the drops were administered. They also observed whether or not the numbers of polio cases were rising to the levels of previous epidemic years. Then they monitored children who had received the vaccine for paralysis and other side effects. The conclusion of the trial was that the vaccine was both safe and effective. Dorothy Horstmann of Yale University, who observed the trials as an independent expert largely agreed with the Soviet assessment. 'Extensive mass programs of poliomyelitis vaccination using Sabin's strains of the virus have been carried out in the USSR, beginning in January 1959. To date, some 10 to 15 million persons have been vaccinated. The evidence seems conclusive that these strains are safe, both to vaccines and their communities…The marked reduction of cases in 1959 in orally vaccinated Republics suggest that the vaccine may have played a significant role in reducing the incidence of paralytic poliomyelitis'.[18]

After reviewing the trial results at the end of 1959, Soviet health authorities decided to switch entirely to the Sabin vaccine from the Salk vaccine becoming the first country in the world to do so. By the first three months of 1960, another 50 million doses had been administered to children in the USSR. Yet while the Soviet trials paved the way for the eventual use of the Sabin vaccine in the United States, there was a more significant advance in a different part of the world for the campaign to eradicate polio globally. These were the trials conducted in the town of Toluca in Mexico in 1958 and 1959, by Manuel Ramos Alvarez, a Mexican physician who had worked closely with Sabin in Cincinnati.

Toluca was a poor town in Mexico, with standards of hygiene and sanitation that approximated many of the world's developing countries. It was an environment where children were infected periodically from a young age with other enteric viruses, and their intestines were rich with a variety of competing viruses. How would Sabin's weakened viral strains perform in such an environment? Would they be able to compete with other enteric viruses and the natural poliovirus vigorously enough to infect the cells of the intestine? The Sabin virus would be excreted into the environment, and to be really effective had to spread from vaccinated children to unvaccinated ones. This would happen through infected children excreting it in their faeces, or not washing their hands carefully after defecating, and then passing the virus onto other children. So nature, in a sense, would be used to disseminate the vaccine in the environment and to other humans. The real measure of success for the vaccine strains would be the extent to which they could replace natural poliovirus strains in the environment.

A series of meticulously conducted trials in Toluca demonstrated that the Sabin strains could compete with other infections in the children's intestines and cause infection, as well as an antibody response. Most important, the vaccine virus, which was given to nearly all the children under the age of eleven in the town in two doses at a six to eight week interval, caused the wild poliovirus to disappear from the environment. Sabin's weakened virus had the potential to outcompete wild poliovirus, and eventually drive it to extinction. As Sabin concluded when he presented the results of the Toluca tests to an international conference in Copenhagen, 'The results obtained...are of significance to the vast majority of the world population...In such areas the feeding of trivalent vaccine on two brief occasions at an interval of 6–8 weeks ...constitutes a rational, initial approach at eradication of poliomyelitis.'[19]

Sabin was also deeply intrigued by a nationwide polio immunisation campaign Cuba launched in 1962 using supplies of his vaccine from the Soviet Union. Sabin had been unaware of the campaign until he was sent a newspaper clipping about it from Havana. With relations between the United States and Cuba at their lowest level during the early 1960s with the Bay of Pigs invasion and the Cuban missile crisis, Sabin did not get to visit the island until 1967. But what he saw when he got there impressed him and showed him the most effective way to use the vaccine in mass immunisation campaigns. The Cubans were aided by a Czech expert, Karel Sacek, a member of the WHO's Expert

Committee on Virology with experience of using the Sabin vaccine in Czechoslovakia. Sacek looked at the epidemiology of polio in Cuba, which was primarily among children under the age of four, with the highest incidence during the summer months between June and August. Based on this, the Cuban authorities decided to launch a mass immunisation campaign for every child under the age of fifteen to receive two doses of vaccine, the first between February and March, and the second four weeks later. This timing would ensure that everyone was immunised before the peak summer months, which would result in far fewer cases.

The ruling party's extensive network of community level organisations such as Committees for the Defence of the Revolution and the Federation of Cuban Women were used to reach out to every family in the country. Vaccination cards were prepared, and on the day of the immunisation, which was always a Sunday, church bells would ring to mark the beginning of the campaign. Local leaders would ensure that every family brought their children to the vaccination posts that were set up in every community, and within matter of hours every child had been fed the vaccine. This was repeated every year, so that children were immunised multiple times to ensure immunity. By 1967 it was thought that wild poliovirus had been eliminated from the island.

This was the pattern that Sabin would recommend for eradication in all tropical countries. Annual vaccination campaigns to be conducted on two days every year about two months apart before the peak polio season, in which each child, regardless of whether he or she had been vaccinated in previous years, would receive the drops.

Given the increasingly widespread use of the vaccine internationally, it was perhaps inevitable that the Sabin vaccine would be licensed for use in the United States. It was cheaper than the Salk vaccine and more easily administered, and these advantages were hard to ignore. It was in 1962, thanks to the backing of the American Medical Association, to which all medical practitioners in the country belonged, that Sabin vaccines began to be used widely in the country. A new phenomenon, Sabin Sundays, swept the United States, and parents and children would queue up on Sundays in schools, churches and doctor's clinics to receive two drops of Dr Albert Sabin's oral polio vaccine. The Salk vaccine that had generated such enthusiasm a decade earlier would fade into obscurity. Jonas Salk bitterly protested the American Medical Association's acceptance of the Sabin vaccine, and accused the AMA of 'tampering with science.' At a press conference, Salk declared 'I don't know anything that the live-virus(vaccine) can do, that the killed virus(vaccine) cannot do.'[20] But the tide had turned, and as the historian David Oshinsky observes 'The 1960s would belong to Albert Sabin, in the way the 1950s had belonged to Salk.'[21]

* * *

The Sabin vaccine began to be used across the world in the 1960s. But scientific opinion was still divided over the wisdom of using a live vaccine virus that would inevitably be released into the environment through sewage systems and could theoretically regain the ability to cause paralytic disease. Sabin knew that his vaccine virus changed as it passed through human intestines. He had also noted that these changes often produced viruses that were more virulent than the original vaccine virus in terms of their capacity to cause paralytic disease when injected into the brains and spines of monkeys. But Sabin would not accept that this meant that the vaccine virus could also potentially turn into forms more harmful for humans. He argued with great conviction that these changes only meant that the vaccine viruses were more pathogenic for monkeys, and did not mean that they were able to cause paralytic disease in human beings. Monkeys, he argued, were much more susceptible than humans to paralytic infections, and so a vaccine virus that had become slightly more virulent to monkeys was still safe for humans.

Trials had been conducted of other live virus vaccines as well. Hilary Koprowski's vaccine was tested in Belfast, Northern Ireland in 1956, but the trial was stopped abruptly after local researchers found that the vaccine strains were becoming more virulent in monkeys. George Dick, a professor of microbiology at Queens University in Belfast who was running the trial would later describe using a live vaccine as 'opening a Pandora's box'.

The worries about the safety of live virus polio vaccines were aired at a 1959 conference organised in Washington DC by the WHO's regional office for the Americas. George Dick set out in forthright terms the worries raised by a live vaccine that spread in the environment. Excreted virus could revert to an epidemic form, he declared.

'We are ignorant of the conditions under which this change may occur. You may have stopped ten cases of paralytic polio, but you may be responsible later on for paralysing 100 children,' he argued.[22]

Dick's warning was prescient, but in 1959, there was no evidence that live vaccines such as the Sabin vaccine had produced paralysis in humans, and so there was little reason to stop the vaccines from being used.

In 1962, shortly after the first mass use of Sabin's oral polio vaccine in North America, evidence emerged that the vaccine could paralyse children. The first signs emerged in Canada, where after 4 million doses of vaccine were distributed, two adults and two children (at the time both adults and children were advised to get vaccinated) developed polio-like paralysis shortly after receiving their drops.[23] These Canadian cases caused concern in the United States, and the US Surgeon General, Luther Terry, convened a committee to look into the vaccine's safety. Two clusters of polio, one in Nebraska and the other in North Carolina, in particular intrigued the committee. In Nebraska, between 1 July and 3 September 1962, eight cases of paralysis were reported from seven different counties, and in all the cases the paralysis occurred less than thirty days after the victims had received doses of oral polio vaccine. There were no outbreaks of polio at the time, and the strong suspicion was that it was the vaccine that had caused paralysis.

Similarly, isolated cases of paralysis were observed among children and adults in North Carolina, shortly after they had received oral polio vaccine. In all, the Surgeon General's committee found eighteen cases of paralytic polio from non-epidemic areas, where there was strong suspicion that it was the vaccine, and not wild poliovirus that had caused the disease. Clinically, the victims had symptoms that were indistinguishable from polio. Laboratory tests ruled out the presence of other viruses and pathogens that might cause polio-like symptoms. Though it was not possible to prove definitively that the vaccine virus had caused paralysis, the committee concluded that 'considering the epidemiological evidence…the Committee believed some of these cases were caused by the vaccine.'[24]

Sabin strongly disputed the findings, and produced a stream of arguments to demonstrate either that these cases were not really polio, or if they were polio, it was not his vaccine that had caused them. He argued with the Surgeon General's committee that several of the cases did not follow textbook clinical symptoms of polio. He added that even in the cases that were undoubtedly polio, just because the vaccine virus had been recovered from the stools of the patient, it did not necessarily mean that the virus had caused the disease. A variety of other viruses including other enteroviruses were known to cause polio-like paralysis, and these might be the cause for some of these cases, he wrote to the committee and to other virologists.[25]

Sabin was also convinced that the doubts being cast on his vaccine were politically motivated, and that the National Fund for Infantile Paralysis (NFIP) and its head Basil O'Connor had something to do with all of this. In interviews to the historian Saul Benison, Sabin darkly hinted at 'strong misinformation' that was being put out by the NFIP, and spread by the news media.[26]

As Sabin argued, it was impossible to prove that his vaccine had caused polio in a small number of cases, given the absence of molecular genetic tools in the 1960s. Vaccine virus had been recovered from the stools of some of the victims, but this proved nothing except that they had received polio drops. It did not prove that the drops had caused the paralysis. Millions of others who had received the drops also had the virus replicating in their intestines and were excreting it in their stools without showing any sign of disease.

But there was enough epidemiological evidence for the Surgeon General's committee to conclude that eighteen cases of paralysis were possibly caused by the vaccine. In 1964, the committee looked at another eighty-seven cases, of which fifty-seven were described as being compatible with being caused by the vaccine. Fifteen of these cases followed administration of the Type 1 vaccine, two came after Type 2 vaccine, thirty-six followed Type 3 vaccine and four followed administration of the tri-valent vaccine. The number of cases were small given the millions of doses of vaccine that had been distributed, and it was adjudged that many thousands more had been saved from polio by the vaccine than had been harmed by it. Because of this there was no move to stop use of the vaccine. As the committee put it 'the extent of assessed risk is sufficiently low relative to the risk of naturally occurring illness in children to warrant continuation and intensification of the poliomyelitis immunisation program throughout the nation.'[27]

As new molecular genetics tools were developed in the 1970s and 1980s it was possible to demonstrate that the vaccine did occasionally cause paralysis in recipients as well as their close contacts. It also became possible with these new tools to map the precise changes that the Sabin virus underwent in the intestines, showing how the vaccine virus lost critical mutations that had been introduced to weaken its ability to cause paralysis.

The vaccine only paralysed the rare unfortunate child, for reasons that are not still well understood. The oral polio vaccine virus starts to mutate in the intestines of all who receive the vaccine. But it is only in some individuals that these mutations lead to paralytic polio. In the United States it was estimated that the oral polio vaccine caused eight to ten cases of paralysis every year from the 1960s until 2000, when it was withdrawn from use and replaced by a Salk type inactivated polio vaccine (IPV).

The practice of public health, with its eyes fixed firmly on the protection of entire populations, can be curiously blind to the cost that individuals often bear for the greater good of the population. Thus, for the US health authorities the cost in terms of paralysis was a small price to pay to protect the rest of the population.

In 1960, before the oral polio vaccine was introduced, 2,525 cases of polio were reported in the country. Once the Sabin vaccine began to be used in 1961, the figures dropped dramatically, and by 1965, only sixty-one cases were reported. This enormous fall in numbers, made it difficult to stop using the vaccine. The benefits in terms of the large number of cases of polio the vaccine was preventing were large, and the risks in terms of the number of cases of paralysis the vaccine itself was causing, were small.

Looked at through lens of quantitative risk analysis, it was true that the risk of paralysis from the Sabin vaccine was small. Of every 2.4 million doses of oral polio vaccine (OPV) given to children, one dose would cause paralysis. Or put another way, since the risk of contracting polio was greatest with the first dose and less for subsequent doses, the risk was one case of paralysis for every 750,000 first doses. In other words, there was at worst a one in 750,000 chance of a child getting its first dose of OPV getting paralysed by the vaccine. One child can seem an insignificant drop in an ocean of 750,000, a risk so slight that it is barely worth paying attention to. It is only when you consider that each case of paralysis represented a child or parent fighting a disease that barely existed in the United States that the fuller meaning of this risk begins to sink in.

The human toll was particularly poignant as most of the children who were paralysed were under the age of one. It was not as though the severity of the disease caused by the vaccine virus was less than polio from wild poliovirus. 'Most confirmed case of VAPP are severe. In the acute phase about 4 per cent involve three or more limbs or the need for respiratory assistance, or both, and in many other affected individuals significant involvement of one or two limbs are involved,' a report published by the US Institute of Medicine noted.[28] Sometimes, it was not the baby getting the vaccine who was paralysed, but a parent or another adult in the family. A typical example was Lenita Schafer, whose three-month-old daughter Melissa was given oral polio vaccine in October 1988. Six weeks later Lenita collapsed while cooking the family Thanksgiving dinner and was diagnosed with polio that she had contracted from her daughter's vaccination. The vaccine virus had probably passed from daughter to mother while the infant's diaper was being changed.[29] Lenita Schafer was awarded US$750,000 under the US Vaccine Injury Compensation programme, and her husband and child also went on to separately sue the vaccine manufacturer, American Cynamid.

Because these cases occurred in the United States, they came to the public eye, and individuals had the right to compensation as well as recourse to the courts. Globally, from the billions of doses of oral polio vaccination that have been administered over the years, around 250–500 cases of children and their contacts are paralysed by the vaccine annually according to the WHO's estimates.[30] Most parents have no idea that their child was paralysed by the vaccine, and have no recourse to compensation.

Until the end of his life, Albert Sabin would never accept that his vaccine viruses could ever cause paralytic disease in humans. It is a human trait to be protective of the things you create and bring into the world, whether it is your progeny, a scientific theory, a work of art, or a lab created virus. Sabin exhibited this to the full regarding his vaccine.

Vincent Racaniello, a professor of virology at Columbia University and one of the modern pioneers of polio virology, recalled disputes with Sabin over the merits of genetic sequencing. 'He thought that any vaccine associated polio was really wild virus...he didn't really understand that the sequence tells you that it was a Sabin derived virus...so to his grave he thought that this vaccine can't do this (cause disease)', Racaniello observed. 'He was a very smart man, and the only thing you can say is some hubris got in the way (of his being able to see the flaws in the vaccine)'.[31]

Salk and Sabin never got on in their lifetimes, and each was convinced the other's vaccine was not as wonderful as it was made out to be. But both vaccines played a significant role in the conquest of polio. The Salk vaccine removed the fear of polio epidemics from the Western world and was the first step in the conquest of polio. The Sabin vaccine eliminated polio from large parts of the developing world. Neither vaccine was perfect. The Salk vaccine protected individuals from polio, but did not stop them from transmitting the virus to others. The Sabin vaccine was easy to administer, and could quickly interrupt transmission of the virus and bring outbreaks to a quick end. But it was not as stable as its creator Albert Sabin thought it would be, yet it caused paralysis and became a significant cause of polio outbreaks in the latter stages of the eradication campaign. It was perhaps fitting then that both the Sabin and the Salk vaccines needed to combine their strengths in the final stages of eradication.

PART II

THE ROAD TO ERADICATION

5

A COALITION OF THE WILLING

THE BIRTH OF THE GLOBAL POLIO
ERADICATION INITIATIVE

By the mid-1960s Albert Sabin's vaccine, the weapon that would eventually be chosen to eradicate polio, was in wide use in different parts of the world. But other than Sabin, few in the world of public health were thinking of eradicating polio globally. Few scientists shared his confidence that his vaccine could do the job. It would take at least two decades before a coalition of influential institutions and scientists would succeed in getting polio eradication onto the global agenda. Even in the early 1980s, just a few years before the WHO passed a resolution calling for eradication, there was little indication that a campaign against polio was either desirable, or likely.

Global disease eradication was an idea that had fallen out of favour and the emphasis in the WHO and other global institutions was to build strong primary health care systems, rather than spending resources on tackling individual diseases. Halfdan Mahler, the WHO's charismatic and visionary Director General, was firmly against expensive new disease eradication campaigns and felt that a far better way to improve health globally was to spend money on primary health care. Even after the success of smallpox eradication, Mahler was clear that the WHO was not going to change course and look for fresh diseases to eradicate. As he said to the WHO's member countries, 'important lessons can be learned from smallpox eradication, but the idea that we should single out other diseases for worldwide eradication campaigns is not one of them.'[1]

Despite the seemingly inhospitable climate at the WHO, a small group of influential scientists in the United States, basking in the afterglow of successfully driving the smallpox virus extinct, were convinced that any disease that was eradicable, should be eradicated. If the threat of a disease could be permanently ended by stamping out the pathogen, why not do it, the argument went. Donald R Hopkins, an American epidemiologist who had been part of the smallpox eradication programme spoke for many when he said Mahler's statement 'went too far in its pessimism', and that the search for new diseases to eradicate should continue.[2]

Enthusiasm for disease eradication had waxed and waned over the twentieth century. Each attempt to eradicate a disease had been preceded by great enthusiasm, followed by disappointment when the effort failed (as invariably happened). This would be followed a short while later by a fresh wave of excitement over another disease that some in the world of public health felt could be eradicated. Thus the period 1907–1915 saw campaigns by the Rockefeller Foundation to eradicate hookworm and yellow fever, followed by disenchantment after both campaigns failed. In the 1950s, the discovery of the DDT pesticide's potential as a mosquito-killer made malaria seem eradicable by wiping out the anopheles mosquito that transmitted the malaria parasite. The WHO launched its global campaign to eradicate malaria in 1955. But malaria could not be eradicated: the anopheles mosquito was too versatile and adept at survival to be driven extinct. After spending over US$1.4 billion over a ten-year period the WHO was forced to admit defeat and wind up the malaria eradication campaign. Once again the idea of eradication was brought into disfavour. But after smallpox was eradicated in 1978, it was perhaps inevitable that the pendulum would swing again in favour of eradication and that a new campaign against some disease or the other would be launched. The question was finding a suitable disease to eradicate.

The US National Institutes of Health convened a conference in 1980 of some of the foremost proponents of disease eradication to identify potentially eradicable diseases. Measles, polio and yaws (a bacterial infection of the skin, bone and cartilage that is treatable with penicillin) were theoretically eradicable as they were caused by pathogens that existed only in humans.

Many thought measles was the most promising candidate. An effective vaccine existed, and though most cases of measles were mild, the disease was estimated to cause around 900,000 deaths a year in the poorer countries. John P Fox, a conference participant commented, 'Measles is the leading candidate. Eradication will be a tough job that will require different tactics from place to place. The disease however fits all the criteria for eradication, and the technology with which to push it forward is at hand.'[3]

In the case of polio, opinion was divided over whether Sabin's vaccine was the right one to use in developing countries. Though Sabin had tested the vaccine in Mexico there were doubts about whether it would be as effective in tropical countries as it was in the United States and Europe. The final conclusions of the conference noted that while polio had been eliminated in most developed countries through immunisation, it was proving much harder to bring polio under control in the poorer countries. It went on to recommend studies of both the Sabin live virus vaccine and the Salk killed virus vaccines so that 'the relative merits of the two vaccines can be assessed and the most appropriate dosage and schedules can be determined.'[4]

The most pessimistic voices at the conference came from two people who had actually experienced the difficulties of eradicating a disease. DA Henderson, a leader of the WHO's smallpox eradication team observed that smallpox had only been eradicated with the greatest of difficulty, and a great deal of luck, given the limited health infrastructure in poor countries. 'In almost every country there were periods when neither surveillance nor eradication programmes were possible. The success of these national programmes often hung by a thread. It was really by the grace of God that events happened as they did and allowed execution of the Smallpox Eradication Programme,' he said. His colleague Frank Fenner also warned the conference 'global eradication of any disease other than smallpox would be a difficult task.'[5] The comments of these two smallpox warriors apparently cast a chill over the other eradicationists, and Henderson would say that he was never again invited to subsequent conferences on disease eradication.

POLIO

Reading the conference proceedings more than two decades on, it is striking that measles rather than polio was thought to be a more suitable candidate for eradication. The conference chair, De Witt Stetten concluded 'I think measles is the candidate that has the most backing at this time', though he cautioned that international eradication efforts should not begin until at least a few countries had successfully eliminated the disease nationally. Given the widespread use of OPV in later decades, it is surprising to see how divided scientific opinion was in 1980 on how suitable the vaccine would be as a tool for eradication in the developing countries. One participant mentioned reports from Nigeria, Zaire and Upper Volta that the Sabin vaccine had been ineffective in certain populations. The killed virus Salk vaccine was not perfect either as an eradication tool. The solution, many felt was to use a combination of both vaccines. At a later conference Dorothy Horstmann of Yale University, pointed out that in Gaza, where OPV had been used, it was found that Arab children, who tended to live in poorer, less hygienic conditions continued to experience polio despite 90 per cent vaccination coverage. It finally took a combination of OPV and IPV, the Salk vaccine, to stop polio. This was a sound and prescient piece of scientific advice, which the WHO only took account of in the last stages of its long drawn out campaign against polio.

In 1980, measles was thought of as a better candidate for eradication than polio because of doubts whether either of the two vaccines available, the Sabin and Salk vaccines, were capable of doing the job. Yet, eight years later, even though no new polio vaccines had been developed, it was polio, not measles that was chosen for global eradication.

The secret to this turn around lay in Washington DC, at the headquarters of the Pan American Health Organisation (PAHO), also the WHO's regional office for the Americas. At PAHO, the key figure pushing for polio to be eradicated was Ciro de Quadros, a Brazilian doctor who was at the time head of the department promoting universal childhood immunisation. The Sabin vaccine was being used in Latin America, and with excellent results: the poliovirus was disappearing across the continent, and de Quadros and others at PAHO felt the time was ripe to wipe the disease out of the Americas.

Another scientific conference was organised in 1983 at PAHO headquarters in Washington DC, focusing solely on polio, and attended by the big names in the world of polio not merely from the United States, but from China, India the Middle East and Latin America.

Once again, the experience from the developing countries seemed to indicate that Sabin's oral polio vaccine was not as effective in developing countries as in the developed world. Jacob John was a pediatrician and professor of virology from the Christian Medical College in Vellore and a pioneer of polio control in India. He presented a study that showed that while the oral polio vaccine had produced dramatic results in controlling outbreaks in parts of India, there was also a rising proportion of vaccine failure. Children were developing polio even after multiple doses of the vaccine.[6] He, like Dorothy Horstmann in 1980, suggested that a combination of both the Sabin and Salk vaccines would have to be used to bring polio under control.

It was only in Latin America that there was confidence in the oral polio vaccine, based on local experience. Rodolfo Rodriguez Cruz, Cuba's National Director of Epidemiology, showed dramatic charts indicating the disappearance of paralytic polio from Cuba in less then ten years after annual mass campaigns with the Sabin vaccine. Joao Baptista Risi, Brazil's Secretary for Health, explained how Brazil had brought the average number of cases in his country from around 2,330 a year during 1975–1980 to around 122 in 1981.

The consensus at the 1983 conference was that polio eradication would be tough, given the weaknesses in existing vaccines, and the poor quality of health systems and hygiene and sanitation in the developing world. It would require extremely high levels of immunisation in poor countries, and there was no guarantee that they would be able to achieve this. Instead, countries should begin vaccinating children against polio and bring the number of cases worldwide down to small numbers. Once polio was brought under control this way, eradication could be considered.

As chair of the conference, Frederick Robbins summed up, 'Thus it would seem that a practical and potentially feasible goal is worldwide control of paralytic poliomyelitis within this century, but global eradication as the ultimate goal should not be abandoned.'[7]

But despite scientific scepticism at the 1983 conference, within five years a determined coalition of public and private organisations had persuaded the world to launch a global campaign to eradicate polio. PAHO was a driving force in the push for eradication. UNICEF, the UN children's organisation, and the US Centers for Diseases Control, were willing partners, as was a new entrant into the world of global public health, Rotary International, a club that had been formed at the beginning of the twentieth century by Paul Harris, a Chicago lawyer to promote 'fellowship and community', but had grown rapidly from its US roots to become a global organisation of businessmen and professionals.

Public health decisions are often presented as impersonal science based decisions, but they are more often than not the work of a few key individuals who believe in a cause and are willing to campaign and push for its adoption. In the case of polio eradication, it was Ciro de Quadros, the Brazilian epidemiologist working at PAHO who was the key figure in building a coalition for polio eradication in the Americas.

* * *

On a bright, wintry February morning in 2013, just days after a severe snowstorm had shut down much of the East Coast, I sat with Ciro de Quadros in his large office at the Sabin Vaccine Institute in Washington DC. I was there to talk about how polio eradication had got onto the global agenda despite the anti-eradication mood at WHO headquarters, and the fact that the scientific consensus held that the suitable vaccines did not exist to eradicate polio.

Ciro, as he was universally known, had cut his teeth fighting smallpox: first in remote provinces of his native Brazil, and later in Ethiopia, trudging through deserts and hills in search of smallpox cases. There are photographs of him in Ethiopia, long-haired and bearded, his face weather-beaten, a hunter in search of the smallpox virus. Now, the hair has been reduced to silver strands and the beard is grey and carefully trimmed as befits a respected senior citizen in the world of public health. He was in his early seventies when I met him, but still active in public health, running campaigns from the Sabin Institute to improve access to childhood vaccines. He was also a member of the Independent Monitoring Board established by the WHO to oversee the faltering polio eradication campaign.

After the smallpox campaign de Quadros joined PAHO where he was put in charge of the Expanded Programme of Immunisation (EPI), which aimed to vaccinate children against common childhood diseases.

Polio was one of the diseases targeted by the EPI, and de Quadros saw polio eradication as a simple and logical extension of the vaccination that was already being carried out.

De Quadros was a firm and unapologetic believer in disease eradication. 'If a disease can be eradicated, it should be eradicated, pure and simple,' he told me.

I asked him about the scientific doubts that had been expressed at the 1983 conference (which he had helped organise) about whether polio could be eradicated given the limitations of the two vaccines that were available. He dismissed the conference conclusions as being 'very wishy washy, scientific knowledge was very limited (at the time)'. De Quadros was a practical man for whom evidence on the ground spoke louder than scientific doubts. He was convinced that the practical success in reducing polio in Latin America using the Sabin vaccine was more than enough to demonstrate that polio was eradicable.

'We knew polio was eradicable...we had the experience in Cuba and many countries in the Americas.'

By the early 1980s, polio had been eliminated from a large part of the Americas following mass immunisation campaigns. In the region as a whole, polio had disappeared from Cuba, the United States, Canada, the Caribbean, and was present only in pockets in Mexico, Brazil, Bolivia and a few Central American countries. Completely eliminating the disease from the region through intensive vaccination seemed a logical step, and once the region was free from polio, pushing for global eradication was necessary. As de Quadros put it 'if the rest of the world does not do it, the efforts of the Americas is a waste'. This was because the region would have to continue vaccinating against polio to protect against the disease being imported from parts of the world where it still existed.

Ciro de Quadros' response to scientific doubts illuminate the tension that often exists between practitioners of public health in a rough and tumble world where vaccination targets needed to be met through whatever means possible, and the world of science. For de Quadros, as for many others in the field of disease eradication and control, public health was all about protecting people from disease by any means possible, and using sound management practices to ensure that campaigns were well executed, without being distracted by 'wishy washy' scientific findings.

Public health practitioners take great pride in basing their work on science, but the practical necessity of getting a job done, often leads to scientific uncertainty being underplayed or swept aside. In the case of polio eradication this was nowhere more evident than in the decision to use Sabin's vaccine as the sole tool in the drive for eradication. This was despite the fact that there was uncertainty about how well it would perform in tropical settings, and also about whether the vaccine virus was stable enough not to revert to a disease-causing state.

De Quadros was a shrewd and experienced practitioner in aspects of public health that are never taught in medical schools and for which there are no textbooks. He was adept at building alliances and coalitions to advance a cause and lobbying and negotiating with those in power to ensure the success of a campaign.

He and others put these skills to good use at PAHO to create the foundations of what would later become the Global Polio Eradication Initiative. An early member of this coalition was UNICEF, the United Nations organisation charged with children's health. The first step towards bringing UNICEF on board was taken at a meeting at PAHO headquarters with James P Grant, then head of UNICEF.

UNICEF and WHO were partners in the Expanded Programme on Immunisation, or EPI, that had been launched in the late 1979 to immunise the world's children against a set of common, vaccine preventable diseases. These were diphtheria, whooping cough, tetanus, measles, polio and tuberculosis. The programme was doing well in Latin America where around 70 to 80 per cent of children in most countries were immunised. However, the region was still falling short of the universal immunisation target that had been set for 1990. It was in this context that Grant had come from UNICEF to meet Carlyle de Macedo, the head of PAHO in December 1984. Grant, perhaps one of the most influential leaders in UNICEF's history, had made a 'child survival revolution' the centrepiece of UNICEF's work, and was hoping to drastically reduce the 15 million child deaths that occurred every year from preventable causes. His methods included promoting low cost interventions such as breastfeeding and access to routine childhood vaccination. Reaching the universal vaccination target was key to the revolution he was trying to promote, Grant was looking for ways to make sure this was achieved by 1990.

De Quadros was called into the meeting and asked for his views. He made a strategically astute response that combined his belief that an eradicable disease should be eradicated and not remain a plague for future generations, with the wider goals of the EPI. He told Grant and Carlyle de Macedo that if there was an immunisation campaign built around a 'banner disease' to capture public attention and create enthusiasm for childhood vaccination, then universal immunisation could be achieved. Polio could be such a banner disease, and a campaign to rid the Americas of polio would excite governments and the public and create a wave of enthusiasm for childhood vaccination in general.

Grant questioned whether it would be possible to get the level of resources that would be needed to get rid of polio in the Americas. De Quadros responded that the key would be to bring together a coalition of people and organisations to support the initiative. The meeting ended then, but de Quadros wrote, 'I left Carlyle's office with the feeling that finally momentum was building towards a broad-based polio eradication campaign.'[8]

The WHO's regional office for the Americas has more often than not led the way in launching regional disease eradication campaigns, with the WHO headquarters in Geneva and the other regional offices following up later. This was the case with smallpox, yaws and malaria, where Fred Soper, PAHO's first director had launched regional elimination initiatives that later helped push the WHO to launch global initiatives. De Quadros and his boss Carlyle de Macedo decided to follow a similar path with polio.

After the meeting with Grant, de Quadros set about putting together a group of partners who would contribute money as well as other resources to a regional polio campaign. With his boss's backing, de Quadros cut through many of the bureaucratic procedures that normally accompany a major disease fighting initiative. The normal procedure in the WHO and its regional offices to introduce big, new initiatives is for the organisation's governing bodies and member countries to first debate and agree on them before they are announced. In this case Carlyle de Macedo and de Quadros called a press conference to announce the initiative, before the member countries had formally agreed on it. They had prepared the groundwork well with the key countries in the region, and were confident that there would be no opposition. Most important of all, they had the backing of UNICEF, a pledge of money from Rotary International and the support of a key funding organisation, the Inter-American Development Bank.

On 14 May 1985, barely five months after the meeting with James Grant of UNICEF where the idea of having polio as a banner disease to push immunisation was first discussed, Carlyle de Macedo called a press conference at PAHO's headquarters on 23rd street in Washington DC. Here he issued a challenge for polio to be eradicated from the Americas by 1990. 'We are proposing that the Member countries of PAHO be supported by all of us to achieve the eradication of polio. The time has come for us to say that it is unacceptable for any child in the Americas to suffer from polio.' The PAHO director described polio elimination as a tool to boost universal immunisation against childhood diseases. 'The drive to eliminate polio will be the vehicle that will carry the nations of the hemisphere towards the EPI goals of universal immunisation against childhood diseases by 1990.'

Their confidence that it was possible to achieve this target was based on the success of recent polio immunisation campaigns in Brazil. The Brazilian model followed the pattern that had been established in Cuba and other parts of South America. Instead of children receiving their polio drops along with their other childhood vaccinations, on two days of the year—held six to eight weeks apart—polio vaccine would be taken house-to-house to every child in the country. Over 300,000 volunteers were mobilised to administer drops to approximately 20 million children at over 90,000 vaccination sites. The results were impressive: from an average of 2,330 cases a year during 1975–1980, the number had come down to 122 cases in 1981, after the campaign was launched. De Quadros had little reason to think that the few remaining endemic pockets of polio in Latin American could be not be tackled within a matter of years. 'The whole of the Caribbean was free, the southern cone was free, some countries in central America were free, the United States and Canada were free, so it was just a push to get that final coverage…basically, Mexico, Brazil, and Bolivia,' he recalled.

The announcement of the drive to eliminate polio from the region was a landmark in shifting the public health pendulum back towards disease eradication. It was appropriate that the press conference was attended by a *Who's Who* of the world of polio. This included Albert Sabin and Jonas Salk, and Fredrick Robbins and Thomas Weller, who had won a Nobel prize for demonstrating that the poliovirus could be grown in labs in tissue culture and greatly simplified vaccine development. Sabin, typically, had initially refused to attend when he heard that Salk was going to be there. 'Why is he being invited as well?' he asked de Quadros. 'I am not coming then.' Yet he eventually relented not wanting to miss the launch of a campaign that he had long championed.

A grainy, black and white photograph taken at the time of the key figures at the launch shows a number of well-known faces in the world of public health. It includes de Quadros, James Grant of UNICEF, Carlyle de Macedo of PAHO and William Foege of the Task Force for Child Survival. Standing prominently next to Carlyle de Macedo was a figure little known to the general public, but whose organisation would be vital to getting global eradication going. His name was Carlos Canseco, the president of Rotary International.

* * *

During the second week of June 2017 I found myself at the Georgia Convention Centre in Atlanta, a cavernous complex of meeting rooms, food outlets and exhibition halls linked by snaking passageways and networks of escalators zig zagging up and down the Centre's multiple levels. I was surrounded by Rotarians, nearly 40,000 of them, from every nook and corner of the world, from Coimbatore in India to Accra in Ghana to Jacksonville in Florida. Many were dressed in their national clothes, and to stand at the top of an escalator in the conference centre and look down was to be confronted with an ever-changing panorama. Women from Nigeria were magnificently gowned and turbaned in shades of green and ochre, while men from the Andes wore hats and jackets embroidered in bright scarlet and lime green. Meanwhile men from the heartlands of the United States were dressed invariably in blazers, polo shirts and trousers in shades of khaki. But under the camouflage of costume, there was a sameness: these were all solid pillars of their communities: businessmen, lawyers, accountants, doctors and teachers. Rotary had allowed them to belong to something bigger than their communities. They were part of an organisation that has transformed from a network of businessmen's clubs dotted across middle America to an important player in the world of global public health.

Bill Gates had flown to Atlanta to address them, and a select few would also have lunch with him. The incoming head of the World Health Organisation, the Ethiopian Tedros Ghebreyesus had flown in to speak at a small breakout session, as had Marie-Claude Bibeau, the Canadian Minister for International Development. A European Commissioner, and the Japanese Prime Minister sent video messages to Rotarians. The air of Davos, where the World Economic Forum hosts its annual gathering of the famous and powerful, permeated the Georgia Convention Centre.

Rotary has come a long way from its origins in Chicago. In 1905 a local lawyer named Paul Harris founded a club with four of his friends as the first members, where businessmen and professionals could meet to 'promote understanding and fellowship.' The main reason for its transformation from a network of local clubs into a global player, standing shoulder to shoulder with the WHO, UNICEF, the US CDC and the Gates Foundation, has been its role in the Global Polio Eradication Initiative. Its active involvement as a founding member of the drive for polio eradication has in turn led to involvement with other UN organisations such as the World Food Programme. 'We are at the top table because of polio,' remarked Carol Pandak, Rotary's long-standing representative on the Global Polio Eradication Initiative.[9]

Rotary was a key ingredient in the launching of the GPEI. Without the money Rotary was able to raise, a global eradication campaign would never have got off the ground. But the road to the top table in global public health was long and rocky. It was marked by differences of opinion both within Rotary and without, as initial rebuffs were issued by the WHO, who saw the Rotary as an organisation of amateur do gooders who had no experience in global health.

Rotary's transformation from a network of individual clubs active in their own communities to an organisation tackling issues on a global scale began in the 1970s, as the organisation approached its 75th anniversary. An Australian businessman, Clem Renouf, who was President of Rotary International in 1978–79, proposed the idea of launching a Health, Hunger, Humanity, or 3-H programme. Through this Rotarians would volunteer their skills and time to help address basic issues of poverty and health in countries all over the world. One of the first projects under the 3-H programme was a polio immunisation campaign in the Philippines. Rotary committed US$760,000 to help buy and distribute oral polio vaccine for the campaign.

This early project showed that polio immunisation projects were ideally suited to the kind of work with which Rotarians wanted to be involved. Since polio drops required no technical expertise to administer, Rotarians from wealthy countries could travel to poorer countries and get involved by vaccinating children. This often proved to be a transformative experience. Rotarians who had been involved in these projects would go back home and become active advocates and fundraisers for polio immunisation. 'It was important that polio immunisation was something that Rotarians could actually go and do. People from Norway for example could go and give the vaccine in India, and that was important in keeping Rotary members engaged. They would have these life changing experiences and then go and speak to their fellow Rotarians,' explained Pandak.

Similar polio vaccination projects were launched in Cambodia, Haiti, Morocco and Sierra Leone, when in the early 1980s, suggestions were solicited from Rotary members for new service-oriented projects. John Sever, a Rotarian who was then head of the infectious diseases branch at the US National Institutes for Health, suggested that Rotary should immunise children all over the world and eradicate polio by the year 2005, Rotary's centenary. Polio, he thought, fit Rotary's requirements for a big global project perfectly. 'It (the vaccine) was easy to administer, it could be administered orally, and so introducing this to other countries where there was no immunisation going on, and that was true of about half the countries in the world, was easy. It was cheap—at the time it was about four cents a dose—so that funding of it was possible.[10]

It was an added advantage that polio had resonance in the United States. Rotarians were familiar with the oral vaccine and had memories of being vaccinated, or taking their children to get vaccinated. The fear caused by polio just decades ago was still fresh in people's minds.

So Sever's proposal was accepted and the Rotary Board of Directors set a goal of 'immunising all the world's children against polio by the time of the 100th anniversary of Rotary International in the year 2005.' Immunising all the world's children against polio would eradicate the poliovirus, and Rotary International can well claim to have been the first among all the polio partners to have thought of wiping it out worldwide.

Sever had made a simple financial calculation. The oral polio vaccine was cheap at around 4 US cents a dose. If 100 million newborns were to be given six doses at this price for five years, it would cost US$120 million. Since the target date for completion was 2005, this would give Rotarians around twenty years to raise the amount, or US$6 million a year, a figure that was thought feasible.

Rotary would end up spending around ten times that amount, for a campaign that would grind on well beyond 2005. No one in Rotary foresaw the magnitude of the challenge they were taking on. One prominent Rotarian involved in decision making at that time, Cliff Dochterman, would later comment 'If we'd realized all the complexity, that decision would never have been made.'[11]

Yet for one person, Rotary's plans seemed to be a fulfilment of all that he had worked for: Albert Sabin. Sabin, now in his late 70s, in indifferent health and in pain due to calcification in his spine, had lost none of his belief that his vaccine was destined to be meant to wipe out polio globally. Through Rotary, he might finally have the opportunity of using a disciplined volunteer force to deliver his drops to every child in the world of fixed national immunisation days.

Sever had brought Sabin onto a committee to plan Rotary's polio campaign, the Polio 2005 committee. In typical fashion Sabin produced an ambitious plan for Rotary to create an international task force on immunisation. This was to be an army of volunteers guided by public health experts who would help poorer countries organise and conduct national immunisation days to deliver polio vaccine to children.

The idea Sabin was proposing through Rotary immediately ran into opposition at the World Health Organisation. The WHO, as we have seen, was moving away from the idea of tackling individual diseases one at a time. Under its Danish Director General Halfdan Mahler, the organisation was focusing on strengthening health services in countries to deliver a variety of interventions. And the WHO's flagship programme was the Expanded Programme of Immunisation (EPI) which aimed to immunise children against six common childhood diseases by 1990.

The last thing the WHO needed was for Rotary and Albert Sabin to distract countries by suggesting a dedicated programme to eliminate polio. The WHO was particularly worried about the way the vaccine was to be delivered: not in health centres, but door-to-door. The WHO feared this delivery method would weaken the health system overall by diverting resources from other diseases.

This was a point that the WHO would make repeatedly over the course of the next few years. In a letter to the President of Rotary, Carlos Canseco, Mahler stated bluntly that 'any strategy that does not contribute to the strengthening of health infrastructure should be discouraged'. He advised Rotary to support the broader EPI programme rather than branch out on its own.

Ralph 'Rafe' Henderson, the head of the EPI at the WHO, wrote to Sabin discouraging house-to-house delivery of vaccine on immunisation days. He pointed out that these immunisation days were only in countries where detailed planning and logistic support, media publicity and training was available. In countries that did not have the capacity to plan and implement these days properly, the results would be poor, and it would be wrong to encourage them to go down this road. Instead a more traditional method of strengthening basic health care systems would ensure better long-term immunisation results. Henderson cautioned that 'national immunisation days are not a goal in themselves', but merely a strategy to increase immunisation coverage, and suggested that Rotary 'explore other ways to strengthen the effectiveness of national immunisation programmes in both the short and the long terms.'

The WHO advised Rotary to support the EPI rather than try and eradicate a single disease, polio. But Rotarians did not find this idea particularly exciting. Removing a disease for all time was something that Rotary members could understand and support. Providing funds for a general programme of childhood immunisation did not evoke the same enthusiasm.

Sabin fumed at the pushback from the WHO (the copy of Henderson's letter in the Sabin archives at Cincinnati University has irate exclamation marks and 'NO' written on the margins of passages he found particularly objectionable). He was not the only one who was convinced that donating vaccines, even polio vaccines to a programme of childhood immunisation was a waste of effort. The President of Rotary International in 1984 Carlos Canseco, like Sabin believed that the only way to stamp out polio was to conduct mass immunisation. This would mean that every child in a country would receive the vaccine at the same time, building a wall of immunity against the poliovirus. On the other hand, vaccinating children against polio whenever they went to a clinic for their normal childhood vaccinations, would have little impact, particularly in countries where health services were weak and large numbers of children did not get vaccinated against childhood diseases.

Canseco decided to directly lobby ministers of health, particularly from Africa to get them to conduct national days of immunisation with the help of vaccines donated by Rotary. Canseco and two other Rotarians, including John Sever, flew to Geneva at the time of the World Health Assembly to host an evening reception where ministers of health from Africa would be told about Rotary's plans for polio immunisation. Mahler, the WHO Director General, and Rafe Henderson, the head of EPI at the WHO had been invited as well to drop by. Mahler walked into the reception, and threw a bucket of icy cold water on Rotary's hopes. He said that volunteer organisations and do-gooders had approached the WHO before, but had made promises they had failed to follow up on. He concluded by telling the Rotarians that while he appreciated their interest, 'we would like you to go home. Don't make this an ego trip for yourselves.' Even more humiliating for the Rotarians was that many of the assembled ministers of health burst into applause at Mahler's remarks.[12]

Rotary's efforts to immunise the world's children against polio by 2005 seemed to have hit a dead end. The WHO remained implacably opposed to Rotary launching a disease eradication programme on its own. Sabin's idea of a Rotary International Task Force for Immunisation that would promote volunteer led national immunisation campaigns was getting nowhere. As an official history of Rotary's involvement in polio eradication put it, the organisation's effort was 'floundering in ambiguity. The head of the World Health Organisation, the one accepted public health authority in the world showed no confidence in Rotary.'[13]

But within a year of this very public rebuff, Rotary had found its way back on the road to polio eradication with the help of two organisations that were more sympathetic to its aspirations. These were UNICEF, the UN children's organisation, and PAHO, the WHO's regional office for the Americas. Rotary brought into play the most persuasive argument at its disposal: money. Thanks to its fund raising, Rotary had the ability to pay substantial amounts towards the costs of a polio eradication programme, something perpetually cash-strapped organisations like the WHO would find difficult to ignore.

In July 1984, just a month after the disastrous visit to Geneva, Herbert Pigman, the Rotary General Secretary, went to see James Grant at UNICEF headquarters in New York to explore how Rotary could get involved in polio immunisation. Grant, unlike Mahler, saw the advantages of Rotary involvement in broader immunisation pro- grammes. After the meeting Pigman seized the advantage by proposing a plan that would see Rotary support the WHO and UNICEF by fund- ing polio vaccine supplies for five years in countries where polio was endemic. At Grant's urging, he would also use the influence of Rotary members to build political support as well as grassroots community support for the EPI and childhood immunisation.

This became the basis for Rotary's PolioPlus campaign. The name PolioPlus indicated that in addition to the emphasis on polio, Rotary would also be helping the broader EPI through advocacy at the political and community level and managerial and financial support. Though Rotary had moved partially towards the WHO's desire that it support the EPI, it retained the idea of a polio-focused campaign. In Latin America Rotary began funding countries that were willing to conduct national immunisation days against polio using Sabin-style campaigns, described as PANDI (Polio National Days of Immunisation). It was hoping to get African countries interested in these polio immunisation days as well.

Rotary's big opportunity came through Ciro de Quadros at PAHO, who as we saw was interested in a regional polio eradication campaign. Pigman and Sever of Rotary met with de Quadros several times in the early part of 1985 to see whether Rotary would partner with PAHO. An early obstacle from PAHO's perspective was Rotary's desire to follow Sabin's plan for an independent Rotary Immunisation Task Force. This would work with governments directly, though in consulta- tion with PAHO and the WHO.

De Quadros made it clear to the Rotarians that they were welcome to support PAHO's efforts to strengthen the EPI, but that they could get no encouragement if they went on their own. 'They came to our office and said they wanted to do an independent programme, and I said no way, but if you want to join our problem, then great,' he recalled.

De Quadros explained to the Rotarians the basic differences between what they were proposing with Sabin's help, and what PAHO was trying to do. 'Our programme is a programme for strengthening immunisation, and as a sub product we are going to have polio eradication, but it's not a polio specific programme.' Several meetings were held to try and resolve the differences between what Rotary wanted to do, and the PAHO immunisation programme. One such occasion was a dinner at the Cosmos Club in Washington DC, where Rafe Henderson and de Quadros had been invited to hear Sabin talk about his vision for the Rotary Immunisation Task Force.

As Rotary's official history describes it, after the group had eaten a hearty dinner of roast beef, Sabin got down to business and sketched out his plans to Henderson. Expert teams sponsored by Rotary would help countries plan national immunisation days during which volunteers would vaccinate children against polio. Sabin's plans had scope for these volunteers to administer other vaccines as well against measles and neo-natal tetanus, but the main focus would be on polio. Henderson repeated the WHO's objections to this approach. The aim of the WHO was to help countries develop their health systems, and support them in creating infrastructure that would allow them to deliver basic services all the year round at clinics, hospitals and other health centres. National days of immunisation would not help this process. It would be far better to strengthen childhood immunisation against a variety of diseases including polio, to be delivered at health centres, where mothers could benefit from a variety of services. At this, Sabin lost his temper, slammed his cane on the table, told Henderson he had a closed mind and stormed out of the room.[14]

This marked the end of Sabin's involvement with Rotary. Wedded to his idea of national immunisation days against polio to be carried out by volunteers, he was impatient with Rotary's negotiations with the WHO, and was also unsure of what his own position would be in the Rotary task force. Sabin was particularly unhappy with Rotary's plan that the task force should report to Herbert Pigman, as he felt this would limit the task force's freedom of action. With Sabin's departure, the way appeared to be easier for Rotary to put its weight fully behind PAHO's efforts rather than launch its own campaign.

Rotary was invited to be present at the official launch of the campaign to eliminate polio from the region, and Canseco and Pigman went to PAHO headquarters in Washington DC on 14 May 1985. Given the up and down relationship with the WHO, the two Rotarians were not quite sure what sort of status they would have, and what role they would play in the launch ceremony. They were relieved to see two seats in the front row labeled Rotary International. Canseco was further surprised and delighted when he was led from his front row seat to sit next to the PAHO Director General, Carlyle de Macedo, with James Grant of UNICEF sitting on the other side.

Rotary's persistence, and perhaps more important, its ability to provide money had brought it to the top table. After Carlyle de Macedo finished his speech announcing that PAHO would eliminate polio from the Americas by 1990, Canseco's response was simple: 'How much money do you need, and when do you need it?'[15] It was the same offer that would bring Rotary to the top table when a global eradication campaign was launched at the WHO three years later.

* * *

While Rotary had to fight, or to be more precise pay, its way to be a partner in the campaign to eliminate polio, it was no surprise that James Grant, the head of UNICEF was present at PAHO headquarters as a founding partner of the campaign. UNICEF and WHO, two sister organisations in the United Nations family had long collaborated on global health programmes, though the relationship between the two siblings was often prickly and marked by competition over turf.

UNICEF had started life after the Second World War as a relief agency to supply food and warm clothing to children in Eastern Europe, during the bitterly cold winter of 1946–47. But in the 1950s, UNICEF outgrew its initial role as a relief agency and began to take a broader role as an advocate of children's rights and the health of mothers and children. This role inevitably brought it into a relationship of both cooperation and conflict with the WHO, the UN agency with primary responsibility for health.

One of the earliest partnerships between the two organisations was the Global Yaws Control Programme, which ran from 1952 to 1964 and aimed to eliminate the disease from as many parts of the world as possible. In what was to be a template for the division of labour between the two organisations in future programmes, the WHO provided technical advice on how the campaign was to be conducted. Meanwhile UNICEF funded the penicillin for vaccination as well as jeeps and other vehicles to transport vaccinators. UNICEF also took on the role of being a partner in the WHO's malaria eradication campaign in the 1950s. As it expanded into the area of child health, it began to hire doctors, leading to some trepidation at the WHO in the 1970s that UNICEF was trying to usurp its role. But despite this initial mistrust, the two organisations have established a pragmatic, if not always smooth, working relationship based on their different skills. UNICEF brings formidable fund raising and communication and advocacy abilities, essential to the success of large global health programmes, while the WHO provides public health know-how.

In the 1980s, the WHO and UNICEF were both headed by charismatic, larger than life figures. Unsurprisingly, their relationship too was an often prickly mixture of competitiveness combined with grudging admiration of what the other was trying to do. Since becoming UNICEF's Executive Director in 1980, Grant had made a name for himself by launching campaigns that both captured public attention and produced quick, measurable results. Mahler at the WHO had made primary health care his signature campaign, while Grant had launched his Child Survival and Development Revolution that aimed to drastically reduce the number of children who died before they reached their fifth birthday. His target was common, preventable childhood illnesses: diarrhoea, which was estimated to kill around 5 million children; measles, whooping cough and tetanus, estimated to kill another 5 million; polio which crippled several hundred thousand children annually; and stunting and malnutrition. Grant's strategy to reduce deaths and illnesses from these diseases was described by the acronym GOBI. This stood for Growth monitoring to prevent stunting, Oral Rehydration Therapy to reduce deaths from diarrhoeal diseases, Breastfeeding to boost immunity, and Immunisation against the vaccine preventable diseases that were already part of the WHO's EPI.

GOBI was a classic example of Grant's strategy to build political and public support for larger goals, by focusing on a few specific objectives that people could understand and identify with. Thus the wider issue of increasing child survival rates by reducing the number of children who died before their fifth birthday, was distilled to a simple set of low cost interventions with which governments and the public could identify. Grant had an instinctive understanding of the importance of publicity and advocacy in building support for these goals, and would carry packets of oral rehydration salts with him in his pocket. He would whip them out during speeches and television interviews to show how a low cost packet of salts could prevent children from dying from diarrhoea.

Grant's desire for quick results often brought him into conflict with Mahler. UNICEF was a fully signed up partner of Mahler's primary health care movement and Grant was in sympathy with is aims. But he was also interested in quick results, which were essential if UNICEF was to keep the support of the donors on whom it depended for funding. Whatever its merits, primary health care was not going to deliver quick, measurable results that funding agencies could get excited about. So, Grant and UNICEF moved to a version of primary health care that would later be described as 'selective primary health care', or focusing on a few specific health issues at the community level. Mahler viewed this as a betrayal of sorts, and delivered a characteristically blunt and very public blast of annoyance at his counterpart during a speech to the World Health Assembly in 1983. Without naming Grant or UNICEF, Mahler singled out 'the parachuting of foreign agents into …countries to immunise them from above; or the concentration on only one aspect of diarrhoeal disease control without thought for the others'. He described these as 'red herrings' that would divert countries from the goal of primary health care.

Grant was quite clear about the kind of programmes he needed to launch if UNICEF was to remain relevant, and a campaign to eliminate polio in the Americas tied into his larger strategy. Grant had seen that mass immunisation programmes attracted enthusiasm from both the public and governments. Even heads of government who had little interest in health, were happy to be seen immunising children and launching national immunisation programmes. In March 1985, El Salvador's decades' long dirty war between the military and left wing rebels was briefly interrupted when both sides ceased hostilities for three days for a vaccination campaign that aimed to immunise every child in the country. The Salvadorean president launched the campaign by immunising the first child with Grant and the PAHO Director

General Carlyle de Macedo at his side. The ceasefire to promote vaccination caught international media attention. Not surprisingly, other governments also saw the goodwill and publicity that immunising children could bring, and signed up to launch universal immunisation programmes in their countries. For Grant and UNICEF, supporting a goal to eliminate polio from the Americas by 1990 made perfect sense: it provided a concrete target and goal that would in turn help build support for the wider goal of childhood immunisation.

And so this small group of organisations gathered at PAHO headquarters in Washington to declare that polio would be eliminated from the Americas in a space of five years. UNICEF, Rotary International, and PAHO, formed the core of the coalition that would later become the Global Polio Eradication Initiative and operate on a global scale. The one exception was that PAHO's role would be taken over by WHO headquarters in Geneva.

The roles that these organisations played in the regional campaign would be replicated in the global programme. Rotary was the major fund raiser and advocate, UNICEF the provider of funds as well as logistics for vaccine supply, and communications in support of polio eradication. PAHO would draw up the strategy that would have to be followed, and ensure that it was implemented.

The launching of a regional polio elimination drive in the Americas was a crucial first step on the road to the global campaign. Without the example of the Americas, it is almost certain that the WHO's member states would not have agreed to a worldwide strategy. The use of oral polio vaccine through national immunisation days had shown good results in the developing countries of South and Central America, and this was seen as a sign that it would be possible to extend the campaign. The only missing piece was the support of Mahler and the WHO.

* * *

Halfdan Mahler was elected Director General of the World Health Organisation in 1973 after working in the organisation for more than twenty years, first in the tuberculosis control programme, and then as an Assistant Director General. He would go on to serve for fifteen years as Director General and would be seen as one of the most charismatic and influential leaders in the organisation's history. The son of a Danish missionary, Mahler brought both that missionary zeal and a commitment to social justice to the WHO's approach to global public health.

His predecessor, Marcelino Candau, a Brazilian malariologist, had headed the WHO for twenty years during which its focus had been largely on two great eradication campaigns: smallpox and malaria. Mahler had a different vision. He was elected to office as the movement for a new international economic order to reflect the needs of the developing countries was gathering momentum. At the WHO, this meant looking at health as an integral component of economic and social development, and playing close attention to the social and economic causes of poor health. Mahler saw the WHO's mission in this new era as, 'improving health conditions in the developing countries by giving priority to prevention of diseases and malnutrition and by providing primary health services to the communities, including maternal and child health and family welfare.'[16] His vision for the WHO was captured in the slogan of health for all by the year 2000, and found its fullest expression in the Alma Ata declaration of 1978, which set out Primary Health Care as the strategy through which this was to be achieved.

The Primary Health Care movement, in its history, philosophy and practical application, was in many ways the complete opposite of campaigns to eradicate single diseases. Disease eradication campaigns focused narrowly on hunting and destroying the pathogens that caused disease, and mounted elaborate, military-style campaigns against pathogens. But primary health care had its historical roots in the tradition of social medicine that emerged in Europe in the late nineteenth and twentieth centuries.

Social medicine saw disease as a product of social and economic conditions that allowed pathogens to flourish, and regarded the improvement of living conditions as the best way to improve the health of people. The nineteenth century German physician Rudolph Virchow is regarded as one of the fathers of social medicine. His investigation of an epidemic of typhus in Upper Silesia, an impoverished, Polish-speaking enclave of Prussia is one of the classics of social medicine. Virchow came back convinced that the real causes of the epidemic lay in the terrible poverty, malnutrition and lack of education of the population, rather than any single causal agent. His report was a meticulous description of the lives and living conditions, and the devastating impact of a recent famine, in which 'many died of starvation directly; many others fell into a state of atrophy that was pitiable.' Virchow's report featured little on the immediate causes or extent of the typhus epidemic (not surprisingly since even a uniform definition of what was described as typhus did not exist). Instead it contained a stinging indictment of the oppressive feudal conditions in which the population lived, and the Prussian government's neglect of the region, indicating that these were the main reasons for poor health, and the proper subject of medicine.[17]

The contrast between Virchow's way of looking at disease and that of his near contemporary, the eradicationist William Crawford Gorgas' approach to disease could not have been greater. Crawford, a US Army doctor who was charged with eliminating yellow fever in Cuba and the Panama Canal in the early 1900s focused like a laser on a single objective. This was to destroy the breeding sites of the aedes mosquito, without taking into account the economic and social conditions that made people vulnerable to yellow fever.

Measures such as introducing piped water to people's homes so they did not have to store water in receptacles where mosquitoes could breed, and improving general sanitation would have reduced people's vulnerability to yellow fever. But these were not considered relevant aims when the aim was solely to destroy mosquitoes. Disease eradication programmes exemplified a pure bio-medical approach: zero in on the pathogen and destroy it without bothering about the social conditions that made people vulnerable to infection.

The world of public health is a church with many sects and denominations battling to establishing the supremacy of their different ways of improving the health of populations. These different approaches are often clubbed into two broad schools of thought. There are those who favour 'vertical' health programmes that target individual diseases including eradication. Then there are those who champion 'horizontal' approaches that look to improve health by improving social and economic conditions, and by strengthening health delivery systems so people have access to health care.

Mahler turned the WHO's focus from the vertical programmes of the earlier decades to a horizontal approach to improving global health. The high point of the Mahler era was the International Conference on

Primary Health Care held in the Kazakh capital of Alma Ata 1978. The week-long conference, which took nearly five years of preparatory work, culminated in the adoption of the Alma Ata declaration. This called for an acceptable level of health for all the world's people by the year 2000, to be achieved through building up primary health care services at the community level. The Alma Ata declaration was a radical document steeped in the pro-developing world spirit of the 1970s. It was the kind of document that Rudolph Virchow might have approved of, but which eradicationists like Gorgas and Fred Soper would have dismissed as woolly and unscientific.

Disease eradication campaigns were, in Mahler's thinking, every-thing that primary health care was not. They were decided on the basis of global and national priorities, rather than community priorities, they tackled a single disease, rather than a broad range of health priorities, and they did little to strengthen the health system as a whole, since eradication campaigns tended to be one off affairs. Once the campaign ended, the resources to support it were also turned off.

As Mahler described it 'The goal was not to eradicate all diseases and illnesses by 2000; we knew that would have been impossible. Our goal was to focus world attention on health inequities and on trying to attain an acceptable level of health, equitably distributed throughout the world.'[18]

The key to launching a global campaign to eradicate polio was to get Mahler on board. And nothing in Mahler's fifteen years as head of the WHO had indicated that he would abandon his deep-rooted objections to spending time and resources eliminating a single disease, when health could be better improved by spending the same resources on developing primary health care systems. Yet in one of his last speeches as Director General, just months before his retirement, Mahler in what appears to have been a dramatic change of heart, called on the WHO's member countries to launch a campaign to eradicate polio.

So what had caused this? Part of the key to Mahler's volte-face appears to have been a meeting in the French town of Talloires in March 1988, organised by the Task Force for Child Protection. This was a coalition of international organisations including UNICEF, the WHO, the World Bank and the Rockefeller Foundation. The aim of the meeting was to promote universal childhood immunisation, and ministers of health and senior health officials from all over the world were present.

Polio eradication was not on the original agenda and it was de Quadros working deftly behind the scenes who managed to get it included. 'Let me present what we are doing in PAHO (on polio), and let's see what the reaction is' he suggested to William Foege, the Secretary of the Task Force for Child Protection.[19] Foege in turn convinced James Grant of UNICEF to put it on the agenda.

De Quadros's reasons for wanting a polio eradication campaign launched on a global level were clear. He had launched a campaign to eliminate polio from the Americas that was going well, and there was every indication that polio would be wiped out from South and Central America by 1990. But the big pay-off would come when these countries could stop further vaccination for a disease that no longer existed. This would only be possible if polio was wiped out globally; otherwise countries in the Americas would have to keep immunising children against polio to protect against cases of the disease imported from elsewhere. De Quadros had been pushing WHO headquarters to move on global polio eradication, but with little response. 'I kept pushing and pushing (for global eradication) because otherwise the efforts of the Americas would be wasted,' he told me. The Talloires meeting was his big chance to put his ideas directly before leaders in global health.

De Quadros felt his presentation on polio was well received by the gathered health officials. He reported on how close the Americas were to eliminating polio and provided impressive statistics showing dramatic falls in the cases of polio in South and Central America, just three years after the PAHO campaign had been launched.

'There was a discussion afterwards, and everyone started getting excited,' he recalled.[20] Mahler, who was at the conference, was apparently also infected by this general enthusiasm for eradication. It was at this point that his opposition to a single disease eradication programme appeared to soften.

In any large international conference such as the one at Talloires, it is not so much the speeches and presentations that matter, as the final conference statement or declaration that formally sets out what has been agreed to. The declaration that emerged set a number of targets for 2000, among them the eradication of polio, the virtual elimination of neonatal tetanus deaths, 90 per cent reduction of measles cases and a 70 per cent reduction of deaths due to diarrhoea. It went on to add that meeting these targets would result in the avoidance of tens of millions of child deaths and disabilities by the year 2000. In addition, it declared 'the eradication of poliomyelitis would along with the eradication of smallpox, represent a fitting gift from the twentieth to the twenty-first centuries.'

The inclusion of polio eradication in the final declaration is regarded as a key moment in building support for a global campaign against polio. But it is important to note that polio eradication was only a small part of a much wider agenda to increase survival rates for children under the age of five by the year 2000. It contained ambitious targets for, reduction in deaths due to measles, respiratory infection and a reduction by 50 per cent of maternal mortality rates. Polio eradication was very much seen as a means to achieve wider goals, rather than an end in itself. Inevitably not everyone at the conference was convinced that it was wise to launch a global campaign against polio at this time. De Quadros, Foege and Grant of UNICEF were in favour of including a reference to polio eradication in the final conference document. But the conference rapporteur, the influential DA Henderson had grave doubts about whether the Sabin vaccine in its current form was suitable for global use.

As Henderson recounted to the historian William Muraskin 'On polio I sounded my warning again. The vaccine is unstable and while we are working well in Latin America...our infrastructure is radically different from (and superior to) parts of Africa and Asia where it needs refrigeration in the field.'[21] Henderson finally agreed to include the call to eradicate polio in the final document, on the assurance that resources would be devoted to research on better and more stable polio vaccines.

So while the Talloires declaration is seen by many as a resounding vote of confidence in polio eradication, contemporary accounts indicate otherwise. It is significant that James Grant in his remarks summing up the results of the Talloires conference did not mention polio, but rather spoke of the raft of measures against a variety of diseases that together would save an estimated 100 million from death and disability by the year 2000. 'Should we meet this challenge, we would have brought to an end the mass death of children for the first time in history,' as he put it. Over time though, polio eradication would take a life of its own, and rather than being a means to a wider end, would become an end in itself.

6

ERADICATING POLIOMYELITIS
FROM SPACESHIP EARTH

For two weeks in May every year, the 190-odd countries that belong to the World Health Organisation gather in Geneva to discuss and debate the organisation's programme of work. World Health Assemblies, as these meetings are called, can be monotonous affairs characterised by turgid public speeches, only occasionally enlivened by behind the scenes wrangling over budgets and programme priorities. But in May 1988, there was an air of anticipation at the gathering. Halfdan Mahler had decided to step down after fifteen years as head of the WHO, and this was to be his final appearance before the Assembly. The year also marked the 40th anniversary of the founding of the WHO, and the tenth anniversary of the Alma Ata declaration. Events were planned to commemorate both occasions, and the Assembly was also planning a tribute to the departing Director General.

Mahler made two formal speeches to the Assembly that year. The first was an annual report in which the Director General traditionally reflects on the year that has passed, and sets forth his ideas for the future. Mahler used this speech to state in eloquent terms his vision of access to health care as an essential element of social justice, and of the importance of community action to achieve health. Health policy should be about 'greater equity and decency in health matters and empathy for the underprivileged.' Restating the philosophy behind

107

primary health care, Mahler also stressed the need for communities to be self-reliant, and not fall into the trap of being dependent on aid. 'People can be carriers of their own health destiny', he said.[1]

His second speech to the Assembly was to mark the fortieth anniversary of the WHO, and the tenth anniversary of his most important initiative as Director General, the Alma Ata declaration. The address saw Mahler once again at his eloquent best restating the case for primary health care as the driver for health policy. But he also listed the achievements of the WHO in its four decades of existence, including the eradication of smallpox, and the rapid increase in childhood immunisation rates. Then he made a suggestion that seemed to go against all that he had advocated during his one and a half decades as the head of WHO. 'What about having the guts to eradicate poliomyelitis from spaceship earth by the year 2000? I think we should. I think it is do-able. And therefore there is no excuse for not trying and trying very hard to do it,' he told the WHO's member countries.[2] Mahler had once famously declared after smallpox was eradicated that the WHO would never again get involved in expensive and time-consuming eradication programmes. Instead it would focus on building health systems and fighting multiple diseases at the same time. As discussed in the last chapter, this was a dramatic about-turn.

The Executive Board of the WHO, the organisation's highest governing body, normally meets at the beginning of every year ahead of the World Health Assembly to consider and recommend major initiatives. But polio eradication had never been discussed at the Board meeting in January that year. The customary route for a resolution by the World Health Assembly was for the WHO Secretariat to make a proposal to the Executive Board along with a draft resolution. The Board would discuss and then approve the proposal and send a draft resolution for the World Health Assembly to debate and decide on. None of this had been done. All the same, Mahler's proposal set off a flurry of activity and the WHO Secretariat quickly put together a draft resolution that was duly passed, with little debate, by the World Health Assembly.

What moved Halfdan Mahler, who had spent his entire tenure as head of the WHO opposing disease eradication, to suddenly propose this new campaign in one of his last acts at the organisation? Again as discussed in the last chapter, the Talloires meeting three months earlier where polio eradication had been endorsed as one of a series of goals to ensure child survival might have helped. Ciro de Quadros, who had made a presentation on the polio campaign in Latin America at the Talloires meeting, certainly thought that this had been a turning point for Mahler. 'Mahler changed entirely at that meeting,' he said.[3]

More broadly, maybe he was taking a leaf out of the book of his colleague James Grant at UNICEF and using polio as a way to gather support for broader health goals. In his report to the World Health Assembly that year, Mahler had spoken approvingly of the importance of setting targets in health and achieving them. Childhood immunisation rates had benefitted from such target setting he said. Setting targets also encouraged countries to apply sound management principles in their health systems, he said. Perhaps, in Mahler's mind, the demands of a polio eradication campaign would help countries develop their health systems. Perhaps it was as a result of knowing that PAHO had already set a regional goal to eliminate polio, and the WHO regional offices for Europe and the Western Pacific had done the same. It would be only a matter of time before the WHO as a whole would have to respond similarly, and therefore the sooner the better.

The department within WHO headquarters that would have to oversee eradication, the Expanded Programme of Immunisation (EPI), was ambiguous about the wisdom of launching such a campaign, to the possible detriment of wider goals to immunise children against a variety of diseases. Rafe Henderson, the head of the EPI department, like Mahler was a firm believer in using the WHO's resources to focus on multiple diseases through a broad immunisation programme, rather a single disease. Henderson and other officials in the EPI department drafted the resolution (though given Mahler's interest it is quite possible the draft was passed by him for his inputs). The wording reflected Henderson's belief that focusing on polio should not be at the cost of neglecting other childhood diseases. Thus the resolution made it clear that polio eradication was not an end in itself, but a means to strengthen childhood vaccination against all diseases under the EPI. In its preamble, the resolution firmly placed the goal of polio eradication within the wider goal of expanding global coverage of the three essential vaccines covered by the EPI diphtheria, pertussis and tetanus (DPT). The World Health Assembly had already set a target of immunising all children with these three vaccines by 1990. Polio would be tagged on to DPT and as the target of universal immunisation was reached, polio vaccination too would reach these levels, eventually leading to eradication.

The resolution emphasised that 'eradication efforts should be pursued in ways which strengthen the development of the EPI as a whole, fostering its contribution to the development of the health infrastructure and of primary health care'. The WHO's partners in polio eradication, UNICEF and Rotary, were requested to support national immunisation programmes in general, including but not limited to polio eradication.

The language of the resolution was also low key. While it 'declared the commitment of the WHO to the global eradication of polio by the year 2000' it merely encouraged and invited countries (rather than making a formal recommendation to them) to formulate their own plans for improving vaccination coverage and did not convey any sense of urgency. The reason provided for eradicating polio was not that it was a major threat to global public health, but rather that it was a disease 'most amenable to global eradication'. In other words, since polio was a disease that seemed eradicable, and since other WHO offices in the Americas, Europe and the Western Pacific had already set regional elimination targets, why not do the same thing globally?

The almost laid-back tone of the polio eradication resolution is apparent when contrasted with the urgency of the language in the resolution that launched the smallpox eradication campaign in 1959. That resolution began by stating that smallpox was a widespread, and dangerous infectious disease that menaced the life and health of populations. It recommended that governments vaccinate and re-vaccinate their populations until the disease was stamped out.

In keeping with the tone of the polio resolution, discussion in the World Health Assembly was also brief and desultory. Canada introduced the resolution (though the WHO staff draft resolutions and are often the moving spirit behind them, only the WHO's member countries can introduce, debate and approve these resolutions). Its representative, a Dr Glynn, briefly explained the factors that had led to it. The Director General had invited countries to set this goal, and that he believed the WHO could and should adopt this goal, three WHO regions had a goal of eliminating polio, and Rotary had promised financial support.

ERADICATING POLIOMYELITIS FROM SPACESHIP EARTH

All who spoke in the debate backed the resolution, though a few made prescient comments about the difficulties that lay ahead. Dr Bart, the US representative pointed out that eradicating polio would be a more complex undertaking than eradicating smallpox. A particular concern was the vaccine, which was not heat stable and required a cold chain to stay potent. Laboratory capacity would have to be increased in developing countries to distinguish polio infections from other enteroviruses, he noted.[4]

The Indian representative, a Mr Ahooja, was surprisingly optimistic, given the problems that the country would face in eradicating polio in the decades ahead. The objective of polio eradication was achievable, he said, even though there were technical problems with the vaccine and ensuring a cold chain to keep the vaccine potent. Nevertheless, given the same determination that had been applied to smallpox eradication, polio could be eradicated well before 2000.

A few developing countries raised the need for technical and financial assistance to achieve eradication. After a brief discussion the resolution was adopted, committing the WHO and its member countries to what was to become one of the largest global health programmes that the world had seen. The programme that would drag on decades beyond its original deadline, stretching the WHO and its staff to an extent that could not be imagined.

The speed with which the resolution to eradicate polio was introduced and voted on without any preliminary technical evaluation is astonishing. Once again, the contrast with the WHO's last big eradication effort, smallpox, could not have been greater. The control of smallpox had been discussed at several World Health Assemblies from 1950, shortly after the WHO was established. A campaign to eradicate the disease had been first proposed in 1953 by the WHO's first Director General, Brock Chisholm. It was debated for two years by WHO members before they decided eradication was unfeasible and dropped the idea. It was revived in 1958 by Viktor Zhdanov, Deputy Health Minister of the USSR, who presented a technical report to the World Health Assembly that year. He concluded that global eradication of smallpox could be achieved within ten years thanks to a newly developed freeze-dried vaccine, which unlike earlier vaccines was heat stable and suitable for use in tropical countries.

After a thorough discussion of Zhdanov's proposal, the World Health Assembly asked the Director General to provide a detailed report looking into the financial, administrative, as well as technical requirements of an eradication programme. This included ensuring sufficient quantities of vaccine and enough trained vaccinators to administer it. The following year, the WHO secretariat prepared a lengthy report that estimated that eradication was possible if around 80 per cent of the population in endemic areas were vaccinated. It suggested creating a smallpox eradication service within the health services of these countries to carry out vaccination, and estimated that the campaign would cost around US$97 million. It was on this basis that the World Health Assembly approved a campaign to eradicate smallpox globally.

In the case of polio, there was no discussion of the strategy to achieve eradication, what would be required in terms of infrastructure and crucially, what all of this was going to cost. The decision to eradicate appeared to have been based on hope and faith rather than a hard-headed analysis of what such a campaign would entail.

7

A HASTY DECISION AND A SLOW START

Many of the problems the polio programme would encounter in the decades ahead, can be attributed to the haste with which the WHO plunged into this new venture propelled by the enthusiasm of PAHO, the promise of financial support from Rotary, and the dramatic change of heart by Halfdan Mahler. In 1988, it was not even clear that the most basic requirement for eradication—a vaccine that would be effective in both temperate and tropical conditions—existed. Scientific conferences in 1980 and 1983 had pointed to the weaknesses of both the Sabin and the Salk vaccines. The Salk vaccine was safe and effective, but was more expensive than the Sabin vaccine, and required trained health care workers to administer it. Also, while the Salk vaccine protected those who received it from developing polio, it did not prevent immunised individuals from acting as carriers and transmitters of the virus. This, it was felt, would be a major disadvantage in an eradication campaign, where stopping transmission was as important as protecting individuals.

The oral vaccine on the other hand was cheap and easy to administer, and if properly administered, worked almost miraculously and knocked wild poliovirus out of circulation. As the experience of poor countries in South America had shown, it was possible to administer the vaccine without a sophisticated health care infrastructure by delivering it on national immunisation days twice a year. On these days volunteers would go to every child in the country and give them polio drops. Yet serious doubts had been expressed about the genetic stability of the vaccine. The Sabin vaccine contained a weakened but still live poliovirus. Scientists had expressed worries that the weakened virus could, through mutations, reacquire the characteristics of the natural, or wild poliovirus and transmit in communities. In the United State, where the vaccine had been in use since the 1960s, it was known that one out of every 2 million children given the vaccine was at risk of being paralysed by it.

Earlier scientific meetings had raised questions about the genetic stability of Sabin's oral polio vaccine (OPV). There were those like Dorothy Horstmann of Yale University who suggested that a combination of both the OPV and Jonas Salk's inactivated vaccine (IPV) might be a better option. The experience of South America, where the OPV had worked well in tropical and semi tropical developing countries like Brazil and Cuba, appeared to have persuaded the powers that be that the vaccine would work equally well across the world. But the efficacy of the oral polio vaccine had never really been tested in the countries with the largest burden of disease from polio: India and Pakistan. Proof would soon come that it worked far less satisfactorily in these countries.

It is also easy to underestimate how vital it is to have at least a minimally functioning health infrastructure in order to carry out a mass vaccination campaign. When the oral polio vaccine was developed, one of its many benefits was thought to be that it could be delivered to children even in the absence of a strong health system. Anyone, after all, could be trained to put two drops of vaccine into a child's mouth.

But in reality, the simple act of getting vaccine into a child's mouth requires a complex planning process. Adequate vaccine needs to be procured, based on the numbers of children who need to be covered (and these figures are not equally reliable or easily accessible in all countries). The vaccine needs to be ordered from manufacturers at an affordable price, and if the campaign is global, orders need to be estimated and placed well in so that manufacturers can ramp up their capacity. Once delivered, the vaccines need to be stored at central repositories with adequate power supply to keep them refrigerated at the correct temperature. Beyond this detailed plans are needed to get the vaccine to towns, villages and hamlets across the country under refrigerated conditions, and into the hands of vaccinators who must have ice packs and carry bags to maintain the right temperature. Where local health services are poorly staffed, volunteers and workers from other government departments such as teachers need to be drafted in. This in turn requires coordination between different departments and ministries, and presupposes a commitment to eradicate polio not only from the ministry of health, but from the entire government, which means the head of government needs to take polio eradication seriously.

If the vaccinators are to go house-to-house, then detailed plans need to be drawn of every locality and assigned to different teams, which requires the cooperation of the entire district administration. This can be a stretch in countries without accurate plans and maps of local communities. Transport and other support needs to be organised for vaccinators. The most important players in this operation, parents with young children, also need to be told well in advance about the campaign and why they should get their children immunised through polio drops.

After the immunisation days, surveys need to be conducted to see what percentage of children have been vaccinated, and follow-up vaccination days need to be scheduled to get these missed children. And then the whole operation needs to be repeated six to eight weeks later, and then again the next year, and every year until there is no evidence that the virus is still circulating in the population.

Being confident that the poliovirus no longer circulates in a country requires a system of disease surveillance that works on two levels. The first step is to detect children with obvious symptoms of polio. Doctors and health care centres are the main places where cases of polio can be first detected. But in societies where doctors are few and far between, or where parents cannot afford to take their children to doctors, it is easy to miss cases. Even when a child is diagnosed with polio on the basis of the clinical symptoms, this diagnosis needs to be confirmed by laboratory tests. There are other diseases that mimic polio such as paralysis, and only laboratory tests of the child's stools to detect poliovirus can confirm the diagnosis. This requires a network of laboratories capable of performing these tests, as well as a health infrastructure that can collect these samples, and ensure they are quickly delivered to these labs. Ideally, two stool samples need to be collected two weeks apart to confirm a diagnosis.

In 1988, in large parts of the developing world there were huge obstacles to achieving any of this. Latin America was the exception. Despite pockets of poverty and underdevelopment, health systems were in general developed enough to cope with these demands. But what worked in Latin America was not necessarily going to work in the rest of the world.

* * *

Resolution WHA 41.28, as the declaration to eradicate polio was formally known in the WHO, was vague on details. It did not spell out which of the two existing polio vaccines should be used by countries, nor did it spell out the method these vaccines were to be delivered to children. The only advice the resolution contained was for countries where at least 70 per cent of children were being regularly immunised against polio. This advice was to 'formulate plans for the elimination of wild poliomyelitis viruses in ways which strengthen and sustain their national immunisation programmes'. Countries below this mark were asked to raise immunisation to the 70 per cent level in ways that also increased the coverage of other vaccines (there is nothing in the record to suggest why 70 per cent was chosen as the figure to aspire to as a first step). Countries that had eliminated polio were asked to share their expertise with other countries.

The method by which polio vaccine was to be delivered to children was not clear. Should polio vaccine be seen as part and parcel of routine childhood vaccination, with mothers bringing their children to clinics and health centres to get their polio drops along with other vaccines? Or, if the Sabin vaccine was used, should it be delivered to every child in the country simultaneously once or twice a year, with health workers and volunteers going house-to-house to immunise children, as had been done in Latin America?

There was little doubt about which method the WHO favoured at the time. The resolution stated that polio vaccine should be delivered to children in a way that helped raise routine immunisation rates and that the eradication campaign should be used as a way to build infrastructure for childhood immunisation. This meant that polio needed to be delivered to children along with the other childhood vaccines at health care centres, and not as a special, stand-alone vaccine that would be delivered on particular days of the year to every child in a country.

But giving the oral polio vaccine to children along with other child-hood vaccinations was to use the vaccine in a way that was not suited to eradication. The only way oral polio vaccine would work as an eradication tool was if it were delivered to every child in the country simultaneously on two or three specified days in a year. On these national immunisation days, millions of doses of oral polio vaccine are administered across a country simultaneously immunising almost the entire population of susceptible children. This blitzing of the poliovirus's natural environment with the vaccine virus sharply reduces the poliovirus' ability to survive and reproduce, and if these immunisation days are done regularly for a number of years the virus will eventually be driven to extinction.

By contrast, vaccinating children against polio as part of normal childhood immunisation has a different impact on the poliovirus' ability to survive. Children get their polio drops along with immunisation against diphtheria, tetanus, whooping cough and other illnesses depending on their age. Six, ten and fourteen weeks would be a typical schedule for an infant's immunisation in the first year of its life. While this protects the individual child, it does not have the same impact on the wider environment in which the poliovirus circulates, since not every child is vaccinated at the same time. So at any point in time there will always be a number of unimmunised children for the virus to infect. Albert Sabin was clear that his vaccine had to be used in mass immunisation days if it was to be effective in wiping out polio. PAHO, the WHO regional office in the Americas, had launched its campaign against polio using national immunisation days, and this had played a key part in its being so close to eliminating polio from the region.

But WHO headquarters, at the time was clear that poor countries should not launch on national immunisation days for polio, but should concentrate their meagre resources on building up routine delivery of vaccines through primary health care systems. To try house-to-house delivery of polio drops, was likely to drain resources from already starved primary health care systems.

The WHO's thinking was guided by Rafe Henderson, who was perceived by more ardent eradicationists like de Quadros as being opposed to polio eradication campaign. 'Rafe didn't like the programme, Rafe never wanted to start the programme,' de Quadros felt.[1]

This view of Henderson being completely opposed to the polio eradication probably does him some disservice, and his views were more nuanced. In an oral history interview Henderson admitted that he used to declare 'I am not interested in eradication. I am interested in long term immunisation.' But he agreed that by the late 1980s, when the polio eradication resolution was adopted at the World Health Assembly, he too believed that having an eradication campaign would generate enthusiasm for childhood vaccination programmes in general. 'I do think the occasional disease specific initiative, whether it is eradication or radical control of a disease can help a larger health initiative…'[2] Henderson's cautious attitude to polio eradication coloured the strategy the WHO would adopt to implement the World Health Assembly's resolution.

The first discussion on the next steps to be taken on the road to eradication came in January 1989, where the organisation's Executive Board discussed a report from Henderson and his team setting out a plan of action. The plan was low key and pragmatic, and divided into three phases: first until 1990, then from 1990 to 1995 and finally from 1995 to 2000. The period until 1990 was to be used to set up basic public health infrastructure. This would include a reporting system to monitor poliomyelitis incidence and immunisation coverage down to the district level. There would also be monthly reports, adoption of standard case definitions of poliomyelitis and training of laboratory personnel and setting up reference laboratories.

In terms of immunisation strategy, the WHO's preference was not house-to-house vaccination on national days of immunisation. Rather it was for a more gradual process of extending routine childhood immunisation of all the EPI vaccines. This included polio to a level of above 80 per cent initially, and then to above 90 per cent in urban areas and slums where higher coverage would be required to interrupt viral transmission.

The WHO had an open mind on whether the Sabin vaccine was to be used, whether a better oral polio vaccine should be developed, or whether a combination of the Sabin and Salk vaccines should be used. The strategy plan called for a 'review of current oral polio vaccine formulations to decide whether changes in WHO requirements are warranted, review of combined use of inactivated and oral vaccines and promotion of the further development and testing of new oral polio vaccine with a view to being able to introduce them by 1995.' But it was clear that in practice Sabin's oral polio vaccine, was going to be the WHO's primary weapon of choice in the war against polio. It was already being used in the WHO's EPI programme, and despite its weaknesses, the vaccine had undeniable strengths. It had been shown to dramatically reduce poliovirus transmission, it had been used in developing countries with limited health care infrastructure, and since it conferred intestinal immunity, it was theoretically a better choice in an eradication campaign. Perhaps most important of all, for an eradication campaign that was going to depend on money donated by national governments or organisations like Rotary, the Sabin vaccine was significantly cheaper than the Salk vaccine.

The tone of discussion at the 1989 meeting of the WHO's Executive Board was in stark contrast to the previous year's enthusiasm, reflecting a certain worry about focusing on polio and neglecting other diseases, especially in the developing countries. The head of the Mozambique Health Service, Dr Rodriguez Cabral, pointed out that while polio might be a priority in Latin America, measles control was much more important in Africa. He suggested that disease control targets should be established not merely for polio, but for other diseases as well. The Indian delegate, R Srinivasan concurred and said that it would be desirable to have targets for other communicable diseases that were preventable through immunisation. The Board went on to recommend a draft resolution to the World Health Assembly calling for, in addition to the eradication of polio, the reduction of measles by 90 per cent and the elimination of neo-natal tetanus by 1995.[3] The World Health Assembly in 1989, the year after it passed the polio eradication resolution, adopted a resolution adding a target of a 90 per cent reduction from pre-immunisation levels in global measles cases and an elimination of neo-natal tetanus by 1995. The intention of both the WHO's governing body and the leadership of the WHO secretariat was clear: polio eradication was not an end in itself, but part of a wider campaign against a variety of diseases.

Money was also an issue: eradication campaigns are expensive, and the countries that had voted enthusiastically for polio eradication were not showing any indication of being willing to pay for the campaign. The WHO secretariat estimated that polio eradication would cost around US$155 million until 2000, in addition to the roughly US$1 billion a year that the EPI was going to spend on other childhood vaccinations.[4] Developing countries would have to raise much of this money themselves. Rotary International had pledged to provide funding for polio vaccine, as well as help from local Rotary clubs for transport and logistics and publicity, but governments would have to meet the rest of the expenditure themselves.

The WHO itself needed money to hire staff in Geneva as well as at regional headquarters to coordinate the polio campaign and provide advice to governments. It had no budget for these positions. Countries that had voted to eradicate polio had not voted an increase in the WHO's budget. The WHO turned to Rotary, which had collected a war chest of over US$250 million for polio eradication, and asked for money for these positions. Ralph Henderson had told Herbert Pigman, the head of the Rotary Polio Task Force that the resolution by itself was not going to lead to much, unless the WHO had funds to hire technical experts to advise countries and regions.[5] The WHO had also sent a telegram to the Rotary International President Chuck Keller, asking for Rotary support for polio eradication, and asking for confirmation that Rotary was willing to stay the course until the goal was reached. Rotary's Board confirmed that they were on board, and in November 1988 approved grants that for the first time were not for vaccine procurement and vaccination activities, but were targeted to helping the WHO build its own eradication infrastructure. It provided US$1.26 million to fund epidemiologists in nine countries in the Americas where polio was still endemic. It also gave US$5.31 million to the WHO to hire technical experts to serve in the headquarters in Geneva, as well as five WHO regional offices.[6]

* * *

For most of the 1980s, the WHO was focused on achieving the target of immunising at least 80 per cent of the world's children under the EPI programme by 1990. Polio was one of the six vaccines given under the EPI, and the expectation was that polio would start disappearing as EPI coverage increased, without need for any special effort dedicated solely to polio. Mahler had retired just weeks after calling on the world to eradicate polio, and his successor Hiroshi Nakajima was preoccupied by other issues including the battle against HIV/AIDS that dominated the global health agenda at the time.

Bruce Aylward, who joined the polio programme in the mid 1990s, and would lead it for over a decade talked about the delay in an interview to the historian William Muraskin. He said, 'polio was not given special priority in Geneva as a special programme, and it competed with neo-natal tetanus and measles... (and there was) tremendous effort to keep them all equal so no one pushed against the others.'[7] This focus on all three diseases was what the WHO members had voted for, but staff who had been hired to work on polio found this frustrating, and kept straining at the leash and demanding greater priority for polio. The atmosphere in the rest of the WHO was not particularly receptive to the demands of the polio staff. 'They believed you would fail. People argued against your position...' Aylward recounted.

The scepticism, lack of enthusiasm and resources should not have come as a surprise as it was part of a familiar pattern within the WHO. The smallpox eradication campaign faced similar internal challenges within the WHO Secretariat. D A Henderson, the US CDC epidemiologist who led the WHO's smallpox programme, described arriving for the first time in Geneva in 1966, and finding that the WHO had given him a minuscule budget. The then Director General, Marcolino Candau was uncertain smallpox could be eradicated and would have liked to have wound the programme up.

In the case of polio, the responsibility for achieving eradication lay with governments, particularly governments in sub-Saharan Africa and South Asia, where most of the world's polio cases were to be found. Governments from across the globe had voted unanimously at the World Health Assembly in 1988 in favour of eradicating polio, and many governments had also endorsed the goal spelt out at the Talloires declaration. But few of the countries that voted enthusiastically in favour of eradication had any idea of what it would involve, how much it would cost and how long and painful the process would be. They only had assurances based on the experience in Latin America that it was relatively easy to eliminate polio using the oral polio vaccine. From that perspective it seemed that three or four years of achieving high levels of immunisation should see an end to polio transmission in their countries, even if the virus was not completely eradicated.

As we have seen from the account of the discussions in the WHO's Executive Board, there were questions from countries about why polio alone had been selected and a request to the WHO that targets be established for other diseases as well. But there was little evidence that countries had really thought through the complexities of an eradication programme, and the logistical, administrative and financial challenges it would pose. The WHO too had not done anything to help a more considered debate or discussion. Mahler's speech had triggered a process that led to a draft resolution, based very much on the resolution that the PAHO member countries had approved for regional elimination of polio in the Americas a couple of years earlier.

Later accounts written by the Global Polio Eradication Initiative paint a picture of strong global support for polio eradication in 1988, based on the unanimous approval of the World Health Assembly. But this was clearly not the case. No one opposed the resolution and a few countries, particularly in the Americas, supported it enthusiastically. But the vast majority of countries voted in favour of the resolution without giving it too much consideration, in the same way hundreds of other resolutions and decisions are voted on every year in intergovernmental organisations, by delegates who have not had the time or resources to really study the implications of what they vote for.

A meeting of experts called by the WHO in September 1990 pointed to problems that would be a constant refrain in the years and decades ahead. It observed that, 'A demonstrable political commitment is not yet apparent in all countries; added resources are required both for the programme implementation and for research'.[8] It pinpointed obstacles on the road to eradication that had not been considered or debated before the decision to eradicate was taken. For one, in countries like India, immunisation levels of even above 90 per cent were not a guarantee of eradication. The poliovirus could keep transmitting in communities with high levels of immunisation because there could be children who had not gone through the entire course of three or four doses of OPV. Even when the general rate of immunisation in a population was high, there might be pockets of unimmunised children through which the virus could spread.

The expert group also warned that if the poliovirus was re-intro-duced into populations where it had not been present for a while, it could spread explosively, even if the population in general was well immunised. This was dramatically demonstrated in Oman in 1988, where, despite an excellent routine immunisation programme that had covered 87 per cent of children with three doses of oral polio vaccine, an importation of the virus from South Asia caused an outbreak with 118 cases of paralytic disease. A study published in the *Lancet* found that many fully vaccinated children were still transmitting the poliovirus to others, even if they were not falling ill themselves. This suggested that the OPV was not as effective as thought to be, even though the vaccine quality was good and there had been no failures in the cold chain.[9] This was a warning of problems to come. Already it was apparent that the OPV did not work as well in South Asia as it had worked in Latin America. These were issues that would crop up repeatedly in the years ahead, as the year 2000 deadline for polio eradication drew closer.

8

IN THE DOLDRUMS

On 28 February 2007, three months after she had been appointed Director General of the World Health Organisation, Margaret Chan, summoned an urgent meeting to discuss a problem she had inherited. The polio eradication campaign was seven years behind schedule, running short of cash, and seemingly achieving nothing. Three Director Generals of the WHO had come and gone since Halfdan Mahler had called for polio to be eradicated, and the poliovirus had outlasted them all. Margaret Chan did not want the poliovirus to outlast her, but the situation did not look good.

The poliovirus was proving extremely difficult to dislodge from its strongholds in India, Pakistan, Afghanistan and Nigeria. And travellers were taking the virus from these places and reintroducing it into countries that the polio campaign had earlier declared free of the disease. Could polio ever be eradicated? Or was polio destined to join malaria and yellow fever in the list of failed eradication campaigns? And how much longer were donors and agencies going to fund a campaign that had no assurance of success? Within the world of public health scientists were also beginning to question the wisdom of an expensive and seemingly quixotic quest.

Two well-known public health experts, the Japanese virologist Isao Arita and the Australian virologist Frank Fenner, had a year earlier published an influential paper in the journal Science arguing that the

WHO should wind up the eradication campaign. Instead, they argued it should aim for the less challenging option of controlling the number of cases globally to around 500 cases a year (something that had been more or less achieved already). 'We believe that global eradication is unlikely to be achieved,' they wrote.[1]

They argued there were significant differences between the successful smallpox eradication campaign and polio. Polio cases were far harder to detect than smallpox since most people infected with polio showed no symptoms. This made disease surveillance extremely difficult and raised questions about whether one would ever know if polio was really eradicated. Another key difference was that the oral vaccine virus could revert to a disease-causing form, complicating the goal of eradication.

Arita and Fenner wrote that it was difficult to sustain the high level of commitment and funding required for a disease eradication programme for more than ten to fifteen years. At the time they wrote in 2006, the polio campaign had dragged on for eighteen years and showed no signs of ending. Smallpox eradication was done in ten years. The world had spent US$4 billion on trying to stamp out polio so far to date, while smallpox eradication had only cost US$100 million. And polio eradication would cost at least another US$1.2 billion, they thought. While much of this money came from wealthy donor countries, poor countries also had to match what donors spent with their own resources. And these countries had other health needs from which funds would be diverted to polio. For all these reasons, the authors concluded that the eradication programme should be wound up.

Chan had summoned the February meeting at the WHO's headquarters in Geneva to rally support for the campaign, rebut the arguments against eradication Arita and Fenner had made, and make it clear that the WHO was not going to give up. All the big players in polio eradication were present: the WHO's polio team led by its Director, Bruce Aylward, as well as the people driving the polio programme at UNICEF, Rotary, the US CDC, the Gates Foundation, donor countries and senior government officials from India, Pakistan and Nigeria, the countries where polio still persisted. The WHO Director General made it clear that the WHO was going to eradicate polio. Failure was not an option for the organisation. 'In a resolution adopted in 1988, WHO member states made a public commitment to eradicate polio.

That commitment has been renewed several times since then. We have a clear mandate to eradicate polio. And I have a duty to carry out this mandate given by our member states,' she declared.[2]

Chan was candid about the predicament the polio campaign found itself in: money was short, and everyone involved was fatigued. The polio programme would run out of money in April that year without a fresh infusion of funds, she said. 'But countries are tired. Staff are tired. Donors are tired,' she admitted. But she assured her audience that the polio programme was 'on the verge of victory.' There were no significant scientific and technical barriers to polio eradication. The only problems were financial and operational, both of which were solvable, she said.

'We have invested more than eighteen years in this and have invested almost US$5 billion. How will history judge us if we squander that investment? Can we be forgiven for not marshalling the commitment, the funds and the determination to finish the job?' she asked.

With this rallying call from the WHO, donors, governments and the other polio partners put aside their misgivings and committed themselves to the fight that lay ahead. In fact, the main polio partners, the WHO, UNICEF, Rotary and the US CDC had little choice. Failure would destroy their reputation, and make any future global health programmes extremely difficult. Even for a voluntary organisation like Rotary, it was close to impossible to admit defeat and give up. Its members had committed time and money to the cause of eradicating polio, and in many ways, the identity of Rotary itself had become inextricably linked with the polio campaign. As Carol Pandak, the long serving manager of the Rotary's polio programme put it, 'It had become a brand issue for us, a reputation issue now that we had invested so much.'[3]

It also helped that Bill Gates had thrown his considerable influence as well as funds from his foundation behind the goal of eradication. Polio eradication, he felt, was achievable and too essential to global health for it to be allowed to fail for a lack of resources. The Bill and Melinda Gates Foundation had been providing funds to the polio eradication programme from 2000. But it was during the crisis year of 2007 that it became the largest single funder of the Global Polio Eradication Initiative. Gates' logic was simple. If polio eradication was to succeed, it would require large amounts of money, so it was essential for his own foundation as well as other donors (whom he also lobbied to provide funds for polio eradication) to significantly increase their contributions. As he said in a news interview, 'We along with Rotary and other partners decided we needed to take this whole thing to a different level. Polio spending went up quite a bit.'[4]

Following the February meeting, the GPEI unveiled a new two year 'intensified effort' for 2007–2008 using new monovalent forms of OPV. It also revealed a variety of new methods ranging from the use of better mapping techniques to publicity and communication to try and reach children who had earlier been missed by vaccinators. This was followed in 2010 by a new plan that was designed to end polio by 2012. But polio still had not disappeared in 2012 so a new 'Polio Eradication Endgame Strategic Plan 2013–2018', was created with the aim of stamping out polio by the end of 2018.

Each of these plans were described as using new approaches and strategies to wipe out the virus. But their aim remained the same: to pump in as many doses of OPV into the mouths of as many children as possible in the areas where polio still persisted. The polio campaign became better and better at doing this. Operating procedures were refined to ensure that vaccinators got to children as often and as efficiently as possible. New mapping and tracking tools were also introduced to locate remote communities where children might be missed, and to track the progress of vaccinators to make sure they actually went to all the places they were supposed to go to. But despite this, the poliovirus refused to go away.

Countries that were thought to be close to eliminating the disease would see sudden explosions of polio. Polio would also re-emerge in countries that were earlier thought to be polio free. In 2001, there were 268 cases of polio in India, and the polio programme was optimistic that it would be brought down to zero in a year or two. Instead, 2002 saw a massive explosion of polio in the northern Indian states of Uttar Pradesh and Bihar, which spread the virus to other states in India that had been polio-free for years.

The year 2003 was marked by a major outbreak in northern Nigeria that would spread to polio-free countries in West and Central Africa, as well as to parts of Nigeria that had earlier been polio-free. Benin, Burkina Faso, Cameroon, the Central African Republic, Chad, Cote d'Ivoire, Ghana and Togo, also reported cases of polio after being declared polio-free. By 2005, polio had cut a swathe across the continent, from Benin in West Africa to Ethiopia and Somalia in the east. Poliovirus from Nigeria even spread to Indonesia, perhaps transmitted between pilgrims who had met in Mecca during the Haj.

The travels of the poliovirus across borders mirrored the restless migrations of humans. Poliovirus from Uttar Pradesh turned up in Angola in 2005, from where it seeded fresh outbreaks of disease. What brought someone from Uttar Pradesh to Angola? Molecular genetics can tell you where a virus originated from, but not much about the humans who brought it there. We do know that the oil industry, as well as a large cement construction project in Angola was recruiting workers from India, so it could have been a worker on one of these projects who reseeded polio in Angola. From Angola, in 2006, the virus was carried across the much travelled border to the Democratic Republic of Congo, where it caused around 250 cases over the next five years. From the Democratic Republic of Congo, the virus travelled crossed another well-travelled border to the Congo.

In 2010, poliovirus from India popped up in Tajikistan, perhaps carried by traders, or perhaps even by Indian students attracted by the low fees and easy entrance requirements of medical schools in the former Soviet Republics. Polio had disappeared from Tajikistan after 1997. But as in the case of many of the former Soviet Republics, once polio was cleared from a country, the health system was not robust enough to ensure that the country remained polio-free.

The WHO and its partners were focused on stamping out polio from the four countries that that were acting as the reservoirs for poliovirus to spread to other countries: India, Pakistan, Nigeria, and Afghanistan. But while cases in these four countries were slowly coming down, the number of cases worldwide did not go down because of these outbreaks in polio-free countries. In 2010 for example, while there were only 163 cases in Afghanistan, India, Nigeria and Pakistan, there were 896 cases of polio from countries where polio had re-established itself. These included 382 cases from the Congo and 452 from Tajikistan.

The polio eradication campaign responded to these outbreaks in two ways. First they introduced new monovalent forms of the OPV which were more effective against Type 1 and Type 3 poliovirus, the only two types of the virus that still existed. Second they urged countries to continue their national immunisation days with these new forms of the vaccine, regardless of whether they had polio in their countries or not. But few governments in the developing world had the resources, or the will to continue with expensive, polio immunisation days once the disease had disappeared from their countries and more urgent health threats existed.

These repeated outbreaks in countries that had been declared polio-free pointed to a weakness in the polio eradication campaign's strategy of relying solely on door-to-door vaccination campaigns. This brought short-term gains: polio often disappeared after a few years of intense door-to-door campaigns. However, to stay polio-free these countries needed a strong childhood immunisation system. Children who are missed during polio immunisation campaigns, and babies, who are born constantly, provide a constant and growing source of vulnerable bodies for the poliovirus to attack and replicate in. As long as there is no poliovirus circulating in a country, this does not really matter. But when poliovirus is introduced into a polio-free country, it attacks sus-ceptible infants who have not been immunised against polio. The only way to prevent a build-up of vulnerable children is to include polio vaccine as part of the cocktail of childhood vaccines that are routinely given to all children. On top of this it is necessary to ensure that close to 100 per cent of all the children in a country are receiving their basic vaccines through a strong routine immunisation system.

The original vision for polio eradication saw the polio campaign as an integral part of the EPI, which had the goal of universal immunisa-tion of children against diphtheria, tetanus, whooping cough, tubercu-losis and polio. The enthusiasm generated by a campaign to eradicate polio, was to be the wind that would fill the sails of the ship of routine immunisation and help to reach its destination.

But the polio programme had gradually broken away from the EPI as eradication deadlines were missed. Progress in routine immunisation was slow, and something that neither governments nor donors were willing to push aggressively. The polio programme was in a hurry to achieve eradication, and its own donors were getting anxious about missed deadlines. So, the polio campaign fixed its attention on door-to-door immunisation campaigns and building a disease surveillance system that could detect the presence of the poliovirus.

But if this separation between the polio campaign and childhood immunisation systems brought quick results initially, it did not bring long lasting results. The countries where polio returned all had low rates of routine childhood immunisation. The WHO estimated in 2010 that roughly 19 million children in the world had not been vaccinated against diphtheria, whooping cough and tetanus vaccine in their first year of life. Half these children lived in Nigeria, India and the Democratic Republic of Congo (DRC). Since OPV is given to babies along with the other vaccines, this also explained why Nigeria and the DRC were battling recurrences of polio. India at the time was still in the final stages of stamping out polio in Uttar Pradesh and Bihar, the two states with the lowest rates of routine childhood immunisation in the country. Pakistan and Afghanistan, the two countries where polio still persists at the time of writing, were among the ten countries that had the bulk of the world's children who had not been vaccinated against basic childhood diseases. Similarly, Angola, Ethiopia, Somalia, Chad, and Niger, countries where polio re-emerged and had low rates of childhood immunisation.

Yemane Berhane of the Institute of Public Health in Addis Ababa and colleagues pointed out the problems in the context of Nigeria. 'Without a functioning routine immunisation service, Nigeria will remain at risk for renewed polio transmission and will continue to pose a risk to other countries,' they warned.[5] The splitting away of the polio programme from the rest of the childhood immunisation system was born out of the logic of a disease eradication campaign. Dedicated teams, working apart from the general health system were required to focus solely on destroying a single pathogen. But the greater the emphasis given to a single disease, the more resources were sucked away from other diseases, leaving children more vulnerable. This was one reason the WHO under Halfdan Mahler (until his last-minute conversion) had been resolutely against launching new eradication campaigns, and had instead focused on building health systems and ensuring that children were vaccinated against a variety of childhood disease, not just polio. In its later stages, the eradication campaign would try and use some of its resources to boost childhood immunisation, but the main focus was always door-to-door campaigns.

It was not just that the polio campaign was not working apart from the rest of childhood immunisation. It was probably draining resources away from it. The focus on polio had led to a huge inflow of funds in support of polio eradication, distracting from routine immunisation. Or as a report commissioned by the WHO's African regional office said, routine immunisation had become 'inappropriately relegated by other immunisation activities'.[6]

Between 2000 and 2010, the polio programme remained stalled, with numbers fluctuating between 500–2000 cases of polio a year. Several deadlines came and went. But through all this, the polio campaign maintained an optimistic front, and assured donors, governments, and the world that it was on the verge of success, and it would only take a year or so more to deal the final blow to polio. Rotary and the other polio partners kept up a barrage of publicity indicating that success was just around the corner.

The same figures and arguments were trotted out to demonstrate the eradication campaign's success. The number of polio cases had reduced by 99.9 per cent since 1988 and the number of countries where polio was still endemic had shrunk dramatically. All that governments and donors needed to do was keep their nerve and back the campaign until the end. The campaign was at the last mile on the long road to eradication and it was just a matter of time before the last poliovirus was stamped out, governments and donors were assured.

But these phrases, used repeatedly over almost a decade lost their lustre, and could not really conceal the fact that polio eradication had stalled. Beyond this, as we shall see in the next chapter, the tendency of the oral polio vaccine virus to reacquire the ability to cause polio and spread was becoming difficult to ignore. At least seventeen countries had experienced cases of polio due to vaccine-related poliovirus. It became clear that in addition to stamping out wild poliovirus, the polio eradication campaign would also have to ensure that all vaccine-derived viruses were also eliminated. This in turn would require countries to only stop using OPV after the wild poliovirus was eradicated. They would need to switch to immunising children for at least five to ten years with inactivated poliovirus vaccine (IPV) in order to protect against lingering vaccine-derived viruses. So not only was the polio eradication campaign finding it difficult to complete its original task, but it now had the additional task of removing the threat of polio from the oral polio vaccine virus.

There was a clear sense among independent observers that the polio programme was stuck in a morass and was unlikely to succeed without changes in the way it operated. Liam Donaldson, the head of an independent board established to monitor the polio campaign gave a talk at the Center for Strategic and International Studies at Georgetown University in Washington DC where, he described how 'an element of magical thinking had set into the polio eradication programme.' The figures of polio cases worldwide showed that eradication had stalled since 2000, and was failing. But, as Donaldson described it, the polio campaign's narrative was in contrast to what the figures were showing. 'There was talk about being this close, to success being within touching distance... the flatlining was regarded as something that was temporary, and if everyone spent large sums of money that were given, then eventually the corner would be turned.'[7]

David Heymann had oversight over the polio campaign from 2004 to 2009, first as the Director General's special representative on polio, and then as an Assistant Director General of WHO. He would later recall a similar tendency in the polio programme to stick doggedly to a particular course of action, regardless of whether it was working or not. Voices from outside the polio campaign, even from other respected scientists, were not taken into account, if they expressed views contrary to what the polio campaign believed.[8] As Donaldson put it, there was an unwillingness to try new approaches for fear of failure, and a reluctance to listen to dissenting voices. It would take a powerful new force to lift the veil that shrouded the work of the polio campaign from outside scrutiny.

* * *

Liam Donaldson, a plain spoken former chief medical officer of the United Kingdom, was chosen in 2010 to chair a new, independent body that the WHO had created to monitor the polio eradication campaign's work. This was to ensure that the campaign achieved the goal of eradication by 2012. Many WHO programmes have bodies of outside experts to review their progress and issue occasional reports. But these bodies for the most part produce anodyne, encouraging reviews based largely on information from WHO staff members. Few read these reports, which are archived and eventually forgotten.

This new monitoring body however sent a shudder through the polio campaign with a series of reports that pointed out in stark and uncompromising language that the polio campaign was headed for disaster unless it improved its own working. Donaldson recalled when the Independent Monitoring Board (IMB) was first formed, 'The expectation seemed to be that our meetings would be small scale, our reports would be brief and they would generally be a statistical digest of the epidemiology of the programme. Instead we embarked on an analysis driven by the need to understand why the programme was failing.'[9]

Its second report, issued in July 2011 was typical in its forthrightness. It declared the 2012 target for eradication was going to be missed, and the polio programme was performing poorly in controlling outbreaks in Congo, Chad and Angola, and it was doing poorly in preventing outbreaks in vulnerable countries. The situation in Chad and the Congo was particularly alarming. Polio in Pakistan was increasing, not decreasing as it should be. And most important, if polio was to be eradicated, the Global Polio Eradication Initiative needed to change and could not continue with business as usual.

The polio campaign had never before been accused of performing poorly. While it had repeatedly missed deadlines, the blame had always been placed on governments for not carrying out the campaign's strategies carefully. The IMB took a much more even-handed approach, calling out governments that were not paying enough attention to polio, while at the same time calling attention to the polio campaign's weaknesses.

There was push back from the leaders of the WHO's polio campaign, particularly Bruce Aylward at the suggestion it was failing. 'It may be a harsh word to use about the programme, failing and it was indeed an affront when I used it the first time,' Donaldson recalled. 'They (the leadership of the WHO polio programme) did dispute it… but to us at that time the present did not look good.'[10]

There was shock as well in Rotary at the IMB's critique of the polio campaign. Rotarians had been largely given a rosy picture of the polio campaign's progress, and were given repeated assurances that whatever setbacks there might have been were temporary, and success was just around the corner. 'The report was scathing,' recalled Carol Pandak, the manager of the Rotary's polio programme. 'There was a lot of who are these people, and I think everyone was a bit hurt at first. But now they have come to appreciate it. The programme was stalled.'[11] The IMB rapidly became a force to reckon with in the polio programme, thanks to Donaldson's vigorous interpretation of the mandate he had been given, and the pithy, readable reports the IMB produced. The reports were a schoolteacher-like mixture of chiding and admonition of the polio campaign for not being able to control polio, and praise when it followed the IMB's recommendations. The May 2015 report for example commended the polio programme's work over the year, and pointed out that this was a 'predictable and direct result of following (the IMB's) advice.'

The IMB's approach to the problems of polio eradication were to look at the managerial and administrative lapses that resulted in poorly conducted vaccination campaigns. It would then suggest ways for the polio campaign as well as governments to find better ways of ensuring that polio vaccine reached those children that were not getting adequately immunised against polio. This would either be because vaccinators were not getting to them, or because parents were refusing vaccine.

The polio campaign increasingly followed the IMB's recommendations, but the story of missed deadlines did not change. The 2012 goal for eradication was missed, as were later targets of 2014, 2016 and 2017. The same oscillating patterns of success and failure that had marked the campaign after 2000, continued. Despite notching a big success by wiping out polio in India under extremely difficult circumstances, the virus persisted in Afghanistan and Pakistan. It was declared eliminated from Nigeria, and then reappeared. The numbers of cases globally crept down gradually, but did not reached the magic number of zero, which eradication demands.

While the polio campaign hammered away at the wild poliovirus, polioviruses descended from Sabin's vaccine viruses began to cause polio more and more frequently. In 2011 for example, when the polio campaign was celebrating the last case of polio in India, seven countries, five of which were technically polio-free, had outbreaks of polio caused by vaccine-derived polioviruses. While the polio campaign was celebrating the fact that that the Type 2 wild poliovirus had been driven extinct in 1999, there was little mention of the fact that its place had been taken by a vaccine-derived Type 2 virus.

The next section of this book looks at two sets of problems the polio campaign had to contend with as it struggled to reach the magic figure of zero cases of polio in the world. One was biological: the rise of these vaccine-derived viruses created by the tool that was being used to make the world polio-free. The second set of problems arose from the political, social and economic terrain in which the global polio eradication campaign had to operate in as it chased the world's last polioviruses. Pathogens thrive in poor communities neglected by government and the rest of society. They also thrive in situations of armed conflict and political uncertainty. We look at the experience of India and Pakistan to see how the polio campaign got bogged down in social and political factors that were never taken into account when the countries of the world decided in 1988 to wipe out polio.

The experience of India and Pakistan also illustrates the democratic deficit that exists in global public health programmes. Large global public health campaigns are launched with great hope and fanfare in the global centres of power, backed by governments and philanthropists. But at the end of the day poor countries need to implement these campaigns. Often these campaigns touch on diseases that are peripheral to them. Or even if they are not peripheral, other more urgent crises, ranging from war to natural disasters push aside these global programmes. Administrative systems are not often strong enough to implement global campaigns. These issues had been apparent during the global campaigns to eradicate malaria and smallpox. While malaria failed for these reasons, the smallpox campaign succeeded. The question was on which side of the balance the polio campaign would end.

PART III

THE LONG ENDGAME

9

ROGUE VACCINES AND ROGUE VIRUSES

By the standards of its own turbulent history, 1998 was not a particularly wretched year for Haiti. Hurricane Georges had howled and screamed its way across Hispaniola, the island that Haiti shared with its Spanish-speaking sibling the Dominican Republic, bringing torrential rain, raging mudslides, overflowing rivers, submerged homes and lost lives. But these brutal storms were a regular feature of the Caribbean, and Georges' impact was relatively muted compared to those that had come in the past (just four years earlier Hurricane Gordon had killed over a 1,000 people in mudslides and torrential rainfall), and the natural disasters that would come in the future (an earthquake in 2010 destroyed large parts of the capital Port au Prince). The country's government in 1998 and 1999 was also relatively benign by Haitian standards. The stunning cruelty and corruption of the President 'Papa Doc' Duvalier years, with its roving paramilitary bands—the fearsome Tonton Macoutes-had been replaced by the more low-key ineptness of Renee Preval's presidency.

In short, the years leading to the millennium were relatively normal by the standards of Haitian history. But one event of global significance did occur on the island. Like the headline-grabbing hurricanes that devastated the Caribbean, this was also a reminder of nature's unpredictable power. But unlike a hurricane's swirling winds and tempestuous seas, this event occurred at the microbial level where viruses rep-

POLIO

licate and mutate, imperceptible to the human eye. And its importance was recognised only by a relatively small group of scientists and public health practitioners with a particular interest in polio.

Haiti—despite being wracked by civil strife and burdened by venal leaders, as well as relying on an economy dependent on the roller-coaster movements of global sugar prices—had managed to eliminate polio as part of PAHO's regional campaign. The Dominican Republic, which shared a long porous border with Haiti, had reported its last case of polio in 1985, while Haiti had had its last case in 1989.

Haiti had eradicated polio under the most unpromising of circumstances. Sanitation was poor and health services were understaffed. Immunisation rates for children for the three essential childhood vaccines (diphtheria, whooping cough and tetanus, or DTP) were below the regional average in both countries. Forty per cent of children under five were malnourished and had stunted growth. And the civil administration in Haiti (the Dominican Republic enjoyed far better governance) was widely acknowledged to be the most incompetent in the region. But in the midst of this potent cocktail of poverty, crumbling health services and dysfunctional government, the Sabin vaccine administered en masse to every child under five in the country over three or four years, had pushed the poliovirus out of existence. This was the power Albert Sabin had dreamed his vaccine would have when he developed it: a weapon that could eradicate polio even in the most unpromising environment.

But this same unpromising environment also brought into the open a dark side of the Sabin virus, a malevolent, polio-causing Dr Jekyll that lurked inside a benign, polio slaying Mr Hyde. This was a dark side that had long been suspected, but never seen.

Dr Jekyll's existence first came to human attention after a child in Haiti was given a dose of OPV toward the end of 1998 or early 1999. Haiti, like many other poor countries, had stopped mass polio immunisation after it had been certified polio-free a decade earlier. With overstretched, underfunded health services struggling to cope with an entrenched HIV/AIDS epidemic, national polio immunisation days were a low priority after the disease had disappeared. It cost money, it took a great deal of effort, and besides what was the point now that polio no longer existed in the country? By the late 1990s, only around

140

30 per cent of children were vaccinated against polio, and in some districts the figure was as low as seven per cent.[1] This child was one of the fortunate few who had gone to a clinic and received polio drops along with other vaccines.

As expected, the vaccine virus replicated in the child gathering mutations, but causing no harm, before it was excreted back into the environment over a period of weeks. Given the low levels of sanitation the excreted virus probably found its way back into drinking water supplies and infected fresh children. The virus had a large pool of children who had no immunity to polio to infect, since wild poliovirus had disappeared, and mass immunisation had stopped.

As it passed from child to child, natural selection, the force that has driven the evolution of life on earth, pushed the vaccine virus to acquire mutations that helped it to reproduce more efficiently in the human intestines. These changes, also gave the virus a greater capacity to harm human nerve cells and cause paralysis. As it replicated and travelled, the Sabin virus also combined with other members of the enterovirus family, in particular enterovirus c, swapping and gaining new genes, and acquiring ever more lethal forms. It also began to paralyse a few of the children it infected.

Within a few months of emerging in Haiti, this increasingly virulent vaccine-derived virus was carried by travellers into the Dominican Republic. The Dominican Republic is wealthier than Haiti and has a much better health system and so it was here this new paralytic form of the Sabin virus was first detected by disease surveillance systems. In July 2000, a nine-month old girl was taken to a doctor in the town of Bonao, about 100 kilometres north west of the capital Santo Domingo, after developing a fever and sudden paralysis. The child's clinical symptoms were identical to polio, and she had never been vaccinated against the disease. A month later in Haiti, a two-year old girl in the town of Nan Citron, 300 kilometres from Bonao turned up at a clinic with identical symptoms. As was customary with any case of polio-like paralysis, stools were sent to a regional polio laboratory in Trinidad, which found vaccine-derived Type 1 poliovirus in the samples. This in itself was not usual: vaccine-derived polioviruses were often found in children with polio-like paralysis. But what was unusual was the extent to which the virus' genes had drifted from the original vaccine virus, and how similar the children's symptoms and the epidemiology of the cases were to wild poliovirus infection. The laboratory in Trinidad in turn sent samples to the polio virology laboratory at the US Centers for Diseases Control in Atlanta. 'We sequenced the virus, and it had a funny sequence,' recalled Olen Kew, the CDC's head polio virologist at the time. It was clearly related to Sabin 1 (the Type 1 Sabin vaccine virus), but it had a number of genetic changes that indicated something had happened. We then got a second isolate, and this time the virus originated in Haiti. When we sequenced it, it was clear that it was related to the one in the Dominican Republic.'[2]

No one before this had seen an outbreak of polio caused by a Sabin vaccine virus that had mutated to a disease-causing state, and had begun spreading and causing paralysis exactly like a natural, or wild poliovirus. 'We didn't even have a term for this at the time,' Kew explained.

Kew phoned Ciro de Quadros, the head of the PAHO polio eradication programme in Washington DC, and told him about this worrying development. A search began for other cases in Hispaniola and soon similarly paralysed children were discovered from various locations across Haiti and the Dominican Republic. Paralysed children were also found in the south of Haiti from Nan Citron and Port-au-Prince, to Port du Paix in the north, and in the Dominican Republic cases were found in the middle of the island near Bonao. They were also found in the capital Santo Domingo, demonstrating the spread of the virus.

By July 2001, a year after the initial cases were detected, at least thirteen laboratory-confirmed cases of polio were detected in the Dominican Republic and seven in Haiti, including two who died of severe bulbar polio. The numbers of paralysed children was certainly greater, but without a system to collect and analyse stool samples the true number will never be known.

Genetic analysis showed these vaccine viruses had been spreading and infecting people in Hispaniola for around two years. Clinically and epidemiologically, these cases of circulating vaccine-derived polioviruses were no different from regular polio. They occurred during the peak season for poliovirus transmission, the paralysis they produced lasted more than sixty days (one of the signs that this was polio, rather than any other form of paralysis), and every other symptom was identical to polio. After more than a decade, polio had returned to

Hispaniola, this time caused not by the natural poliovirus, but by a vaccine virus that had gone rogue. As Olen Kew put it, the cases in Hispaniola had shown beyond doubt that circulating vaccine-derived viruses existed, and they were biologically the equivalent of wild polioviruses in their ability to cause disease and to transmit easily between humans.

Fortunately, vaccine-derived viruses were still vulnerable to OPV: Sabin's vaccine virus still provided immunity against the mutants it had spawned. The outbreaks in Hispaniola were eventually stamped out after intense campaign of door-to-door immunisation of children.

The questions raised by George Dick and other scientists nearly fifty years earlier about whether the Sabin vaccine virus could take on a life of its own and spread in communities and cause polio, had finally been answered. It was already known that OPV could cause polio-like paralysis in those who received the vaccine, and sometimes in their close family contacts: a phenomenon known as Vaccine Associated Paralytic Polio (VAPP). But the cases in Hispaniola were something different. This was not about the vaccine reacting badly in a child and causing paralysis. It was about excreted vaccine virus passing from person to person, infecting large numbers of people and in the process losing the mutations that Albert Sabin had introduced to weaken the virus, and recovering wild poliovirus like properties and the ability to cause outbreaks of disease. These viruses were described as circulating vaccine-derived polioviruses (cVDPV).

For Kew, the discovery of circulating vaccine-derived polioviruses was confirmation of another puzzle he had been working on. Kew had been working with virologists in Egypt to document the disappearance of various poliovirus strains from that country. The Egyptian scientists had virus samples going back several years stored in freezers, which were being genetically analysed and recorded by Kew's team at the US CDC. In 1998, two years before the Hispaniola outbreak, Kew began to find unusual, genetically distinct Type 2 polioviruses. They were not natural, or wild, polioviruses, nor were they Sabin Type 2 vaccine viruses. 'They were really genetically distinct,' Kew said. 'We knew the general genetic signature was for the Egyptian wild Type 2, but these strains were different. They matched the Sabin strain, but they were divergent to the Sabin strain, though clearly related.'[3] As in the case of Hispaniola, these were vaccine-derived viruses that had been spreading in Egypt between 1993 and 1998, and had paralysed at least thirty children.

The Egyptian outbreak demonstrated the surprising resilience and longevity of vaccine-derived viruses. Polio is a seasonal disease, with a low season in the first half of the year when circulation of the virus is low, and a high season in the second half when transmission is more rapid. The vaccine-derived viruses in Egypt had survived and multiplied for at least ten low seasons before they died out, showing their fitness for survival.

Cases of polio caused by circulating vaccine-derived viruses were reported from the Philippines in 2001 where three cases were identified, from Madagascar where eight cases were identified, in China where there were two, and Indonesia where there were forty-six. The WHO at first tended to see this as a minor issue. These vaccine-derived viruses happened only when rates of immunisation were low, and they responded to intensive vaccination campaigns, and seemed little more than a distraction from the main challenge of wiping out natural poliovirus.

This assumption was shattered by an explosion of polio caused by a vaccine-derived Type 2 poliovirus in northern Nigeria that raged for more than six years from 2005 and paralysed over 400 children before it was finally stamped out. Once again, clinical and epidemiological analysis showed there was no difference between the severity of disease caused by the vaccine-derived Type 2 virus and wild Type 2 virus, and both spread across communities with identical ease. The explosion of vaccine-derived Type 2 was particularly tragic because it came at a time when the WHO and the other partners in the polio programme had been congratulating themselves that wild Type 2 virus had disappeared. The last case of polio caused by wild Type 2 was recorded in Aligarh in India in 1999, and the Global Polio Eradication Initiative had held this up as an example of the eradication campaign's achievements. What was given next to no publicity in all the GPEI's campaign and advocacy material was that a vaccine-derived Type 2 virus had appeared in its stead, that was capable of causing identical disease.

The vaccine-derived Type 2 also raised an ethical question that was debated by a small group within the polio eradication. Vaccine-derived Type 2 outbreaks were caused by the Type 2 component in the oral polio vaccine. But since the Type 2 virus had disappeared from nature since 1999, what reason was there to continue to vaccinate against it? Why was the Type 2 component not removed from the vaccine? Steve Cochi and Kew of the US CDC had begun urging the WHO to remove the Type 2 component from the oral polio vaccine shortly after it was clear that the natural Type 2 virus was extinct. 'We were calling it two less OPV,' said Kew. 'We had this idea even before 1999. It was clear that wild Type 2 was going to disappear first. This was the pattern we had seen in the US, and the Americas...and that was playing out globally as well.'[4]

There were strong epidemiological reasons for removing the Type 2 component, even before the discovery that it caused explosive outbreaks of disease. The Type 2 vaccine was a major source of VAPP, or vaccine associated paralytic polio. 'My thought really in the 1990s, was that the vaccine is a source of vaccine associated paralysis...and the burden is going to be sustained indefinitely against a virus that is extinct from the field' explained Kew. Removing the Type 2 component would have the added advantage of making the resultant bi-valent oral polio vaccine more effective: the Type 2 component in the vaccine interfered with the other two types and made them less effective.

The WHO's polio team was reluctant to change. It commissioned a report from an outside expert who concluded that it was wise to maintain the Type 2 component as an insurance policy, despite the number of VAPP cases it might cause. The outbreaks in Nigeria however forced the WHO to confront the fact that the Type 2 vaccine virus could also cause large outbreaks of polio. All three types of Sabin vaccine virus could cause outbreaks of paralytic disease, but the Type 2 vaccine virus was the most prone to do so. Between 2000 and 2017, Type 2 vaccine-derived viruses had caused 777 cases of paralysis in eighteen countries, Type 1 vaccine had caused 103 cases in nine countries, while Type 3 vaccine had caused twelve cases in three countries. Given the dangers posed by Type 2, it was not surprising that the CDC counselled its withdrawal. The WHO however was averse to making any changes for fear that it would affect confidence in the vaccine. It took warnings from advisory bodies including SAGE, the WHO's Strategic Advisory Group of Experts on vaccines, and the IMB before the Type 2 component was removed form OPV in April 2016.

The WHO and the polio campaign never talked to the public about these issues, and the public message was always the same. The oral polio vaccine was safe and effective even though 'in very rare instances the vaccine virus can genetically change into a form that can paralyse.' However, this small risk 'pales in significance to the tremendous public health benefits associated with OPV.'

But this description of circulating vaccine-derived poliovirus as a rare occurrence was increasingly untenable by the second decade of the twenty-first century, as the cases of polio caused by wild poliovirus dropped as a consequence of successful eradication efforts. Yet the number of circulating vaccine-derived cases rose because of continued use of the oral polio vaccine. Thus in 2015, nearly a third of all polio cases globally were caused by vaccine-derived viruses (seventy-four wild polio cases and thirty-two circulating vaccine-derived cases). Of these vaccine-derived cases, Laos, Madagascar, the Ukraine, Guinea and Niger had been previously declared polio-free by the WHO.

Maintaining confidence in the oral polio vaccine was a key objective of the WHO's polio department. So the blame for cases of the vaccine-derived polio was shifted away from the vaccine, to governments and the way they were running their polio immunisation campaigns. 'Circulating VDPVs occur when routine or supplementary immunisation are poorly conducted and a population is left susceptible to poliovirus, whether from vaccine-derived or wild poliovirus. Hence the problem is not with the vaccine itself, but with low vaccination coverage.'[5]

This argument was disingenuous. Studies showed that vaccine-derived polio broke out in areas with low vaccination rates, high population density and poor sanitation, particularly in areas where the wild poliovirus had been eliminated. This set of conditions described large parts of the developing world. And unless the polio campaign was willing to help develop health systems and improve sanitation and nutrition, these conditions were not going to change. They were a given that the polio campaign had to work with, and any vaccine that the eradication campaign chose, had to work in these conditions.

One solution would have been for the polio campaign to help poor countries that were polio-free to build up their routine childhood immunisation systems. This would have meant that oral polio vaccine as well as other vaccines could be delivered to a large proportion of a country's children as part of their vaccination schedule. This was the original plan for polio eradication as spelt out in the 1988 World Health Assembly resolution where polio eradication was to go hand-in-hand with other childhood immunisation programmes.

The discovery that the Sabin vaccine virus could take on a life of its own and replace wild poliovirus as a disease-causing pathogen would have profound implications on the Global Polio Eradication's strategy to wipe out the disease. The vaccine that it had been relying on for all these decades had suddenly revealed a weakness that would have a bearing on a fundamental assumption that had guided the GPEI: that polio would end once wild poliovirus was eradicated. The events in Hispaniola and elsewhere showed that even after wild poliovirus ceased to exist, people would have to be protected against circulating vaccine-derived viruses. The use of the oral polio vaccine would have to be discontinued, and a Salk-type inactivated vaccine would have to be introduced to protect against both vaccine-derived as well as wild poliovirus.

The polio eradication endgame was going to be very different from the end of the smallpox campaign. In the case of smallpox, once the virus was certified eradicated, vaccination simply stopped. The smallpox vaccine had not created its own disease-causing variants, so no further protection was necessary.

This need for continued vaccination after wild poliovirus had been eradicated in order to get rid of polio caused by the vaccine virus undermined a major reason in favour of eradication. This was that money could be saved by stopping vaccination once a pathogen was wiped out. Economic benefit had always been seen as a powerful argument in favour of eradication and a way for public health experts to demonstrate to hardheaded guardians of public finance that this was a worthwhile investment. A modelling exercise led by Kimberly Thompson of Harvard, much quoted by the polio eradication campaign, concluded that, 'eradication is always a better option than control...we should be willing to pay thousands of millions of dollars more to achieve this goal.'[6] But this modelling assumed that after wild poliovirus eradication, the vaccine virus would disappear quietly after a few years, and vaccination could stop. The possibility that the vaccine virus might circulate silently for several years or even decades before popping up to cause disease, was not something that any economic model took into account.

The discovery of vaccine-derived polioviruses that could cause disease also raised a basic question about what it was that the polio programme was trying to eradicate and how this would be achieved. The original 1988 World Health Assembly resolution had asked for the global eradication of polio. Since the existence of circulating vaccine-derived polioviruses had not been discovered, the WHO and the polio eradication campaign had defined eradication to mean an absence of wild poliovirus worldwide confirmed by environmental sampling and surveillance for disease. Polio caused by the vaccine virus, or even the continued existence of vaccine virus transmission after wild poliovirus had been eradicated, would not fall under this definition of eradication. The polio eradication campaign could theoretically declare victory and walk away once wild poliovirus was eradicated, regardless of whether children were still being crippled by vaccine-derived poliovirus. But it took several years for the WHO and its partners in polio eradication to accept that vaccine-derived viruses were a problem. The oral polio vaccine needed to be phased out, and an inactivated vaccine needed to be introduced as part of a polio eradication endgame.

Scientists independent of the polio programme had suggested even before the outbreaks of vaccine-derived polio were first noted that the sole reliance on OPV needed to end. They declared that inactivated vaccines (IPV) needed to be introduced, and that the definition to polio eradication needed to be widened to include both wild poliovirus and vaccine-derived poliovirus.

Vincent Racaniello of Columbia University and his collaborator Alan Dove had written presciently in 1997 (before the vaccine-derived polio outbreaks in Hispaniola had occurred) about the dangers of Sabin vaccine related strains being released into the environment. 'Virus excreted by vaccinees may persist indefinitely,' they wrote. They also pointed to the inadequacy of the definition of polio eradication that the WHO had adopted. The WHO's definition of polio as the absence of wild poliovirus in the population, sewage or drinking water was 'accurate only by a narrow definition', they wrote. The Sabin vaccine virus' proclivity to mutate readily to more virulent forms meant that potentially pathogenic viruses were being released into waste-water and aquifers where they could persist for indefinite periods of time. 'A broader, more intuitive definition would be elimination of both vaccine and wild strains,' for which the use of IPV would be required as well.[7] In an editorial in the *New England Journal of Medicine*, Jacob John, India's foremost polio expert concurred. 'The eradication of polio ought to be defined as the absence of any poliovirus in humans instead of the absence of wild poliovirus in humans.' John also made a powerful call to switch from the oral vaccine to an inactivated vaccine. 'It is unwise and unnecessary to risk failure by continuing to use orally administered vaccine which is infectious and potentially transmissible and which may have reversible neurovirulence. We have IPV, a safe alternative and a superior immunogen.'[8]

But within the GPEI, for at least a decade after the discovery of circulating vaccine-derived viruses, there was an entrenched belief that oral polio vaccine would be sufficient to complete polio eradication. Above all, there was a determination not to shake public and government confidence in the oral polio vaccine, and so any descriptions of the vaccine-derived virus outbreaks was done in measured and anodyne terms. As Jacob John, the polio expert from India who had been part of WHO expert committees since the 1980s described it, 'a religion of OPV' prevailed at the WHO which made it difficult to discuss alternate vaccination strategies, or the use of inactivated vaccines.

The 'religion of OPV' had deep roots in the polio programme. I realised this forcefully when I met one of the greatest believers in the vaccine Ciro de Quadros, the man instrumental in launching a regional elimination effort in the Americas, and a prominent figure in the world of polio eradication. I met him in February 2013, a little after the WHO had for the first time indicated that IPV might be added to the vaccination schedule in order to protect against circulating vaccine-derived viruses. De Quadros, who at the time was a member of the Independent Monitoring Board (IMB) advising the polio programme, was however not convinced that a switch to IPV was necessary, and saw circulating vaccine-derived polioviruses as essentially a temporary nuisance. He told me that the disease caused by circulating vaccine-derived viruses were epidemiologically different. 'The transmissibility is not the same. It does not explode in the same way as wild poliovirus cases do.' He added that vaccine-derived polioviruses were not polioviruses at all, since they had recombined with genes from other enteroviruses. He implied that they were a milder form of poliovirus. 'It is the same as we have chicken pox, which is not small pox.' I was a little surprised by this stout defence of the vaccine, which seemed to contradict everything I had read in the scientific literature, but I held my tongue on the chance that I might have got it all wrong. Then I went back and checked the studies and papers that had been done after the outbreaks in Nigeria and Madura in Indonesia. They all confirmed that the clinical attack rate (a measure of how transmissible a virus is) was the same for both wild and circulating vaccine-derived viruses.

The conclusion from scientific studies was unambiguous: circulating vaccine-derived viruses were indistinguishable from wild poliovirus in the severity of the disease they caused, and in their ability to transmit from human to human. The analogy between chickenpox and smallpox, which implied that circulating vaccine-derived viruses produced milder disease than wild poliovirus, was clearly wrong. I searched the literature about recombinant polioviruses, and found that it was not only vaccine-derived polioviruses that recombined with other enteroviruses, but wild polioviruses, something that had been known since 1962. So there was no real reason for distinguishing between wild poliovirus and circulating vaccine-derived viruses on the basis that one was a recombinant and the other was not.

De Quadros was clear that OPV was the only vaccine that could eradicate polio, and that it was completely unnecessary to use IPV, either alone or in combination with the OPV to protect against vaccine-derived viruses. He based his case on the Cuban experience. Cuba only vaccinated against polio twice a year using the oral vaccine, and 'there is no circulating vaccine virus…they see virus in the environment for two or three months (after vaccination) and then nothing more.' This meant, he said, that after wild poliovirus was eliminated it would be possible to simply stop using OPV without ever having to use IPV to get rid of vaccine virus. 'Theoretically, and I think in practice, you could just stop everything…don't use any vaccine,' he said. Ironically, at the time that de Quadros was using the Cuban experience as an example, Cuba itself had begun studies in preparation for introducing IPV into its childhood vaccination schedule.

De Quadros sadly passed away a year or so after I met him, so the follow-up meeting with him that I had been planning never materialised. But I have often since pondered on why he would consciously downplay the risk of vaccine-derived viruses, using arguments that were not based on science, but on deeply held conviction. I could imagine him, as well as others who believed in OPV, making these same arguments at meetings with the other GPEI partners such as UNICEF, Rotary International and the Gates Foundation; oral polio vaccine is the only vaccine that can eradicate polio; it can have messy side effects, but these are extremely rare.

So strong was the belief in the oral polio vaccine among influential voices in global public health, that even in the United States it was difficult to switch from the oral vaccine to the inactivated vaccine. After polio was eliminated from the US in 1979, the only cases of polio in the country came from children who had been paralysed by the oral polio vaccine. Between eight and ten children were being paralysed by the vaccine every year. This became ethically untenable, as well as expensive, as parents began to sue vaccine companies for compensation for their paralysed children.

In 1995, the US Institute for Medicine and the US CDC organised a workshop to discuss options for switching from the oral vaccine to the inactivated vaccine.

The WHO was not officially represented at this workshop but its strong views in favour of the oral polio vaccine were reflected by various participants including de Quadros. A summary of the workshop proceedings noted that the WHO 'had expressed two primary concerns about the possibility of a change in polio vaccination strategy in the United States'. One was that financial support for global polio eradication could be undermined because the US funding for the campaign could be curtailed. 'WHO officials fear that a change to the domestic use of one or more doses of the more expensive IPV could result in reduced US funding for the global effort.' The WHO's other concern was that if the US moved away from OPV, then other countries might follow suit, jeopardising the GPEI's strategy for eradication. 'WHO's second concern about a strategy shift is that …countries where polio is endemic might follow the lead of the United States and decrease their reliance on OPV before it is appropriate for them to do so' the report noted. 'The WHO leadership believes that eradication of polio in countries where it is endemic can only be accomplished by mass vaccination through OPV, and that a change to IPV in these countries could jeopardise the global eradication effort.'[9]

The WHO's position was noteworthy for its belief that countries were incapable of deciding their own strategies and that they might do things that were not 'appropriate' for them to do. It also believed that countries would blindly follow whatever the United States did (even though there is little evidence of developing countries rushing helter skelter to imitate the high cost medical interventions that characterise the US health service). Beyond this it was willing to turn a blind eye to the paralytic properties of OPV. Supporters of IPV and OPV, like followers of two rival football teams, would get into heated and often unpleasant spats. The historian William Muraskin recounts an argument that erupted at a conference in New Delhi. It was between William Foege who believed that both IPV and OPV had a role in the developing world, and de Quadros and D A Henderson on the other, who were committed supporters of OPV. Foege gave a keynote presentation at which he suggested the use of IPV, citing evidence that a combination of IPV and OPV could work well in the tropics 'Ciro and D A Henderson looked like they would kill him. To them this would undermine the only strategy they thought would work.'[10] Henderson and Foege then got into what was described as a yelling match over whether it was appropriate to even suggest that countries should add IPV to their polio vaccination schedules. The animosity did not end with the New Delhi meeting. According to one account, Henderson then 'played dirty' by writing to the WHO suggesting that Foege was in the hands of the pharmaceutical industry.'[11] Jacob John had a similar experience when he spoke in favour of IPV at a meeting at which de Quadros was also present. 'Ciro came up to me after I spoke, and said I will never talk to you again, you mentioned IPV.'[12]

In India and other tropical settings the efficacy of OPV was low. Children in the states of Uttar Pradesh and Bihar had received an average of fifteen doses of oral polio vaccine, but with seemingly little effect on reducing wild poliovirus transmission.[13] The mucosal immunity that had been regarded as a great strength of the oral polio vaccine was also found to be less than perfect.

Meetings of WHO expert groups such as the Strategic Advisory Group of Experts on Immunisation (SAGE), had flagged up these problems from around 2003 and called on the WHO to plan for the introduction of IPV and the eventual withdrawal of OPV. But there was great reluctance on the part of the leadership of the polio programme at the WHO to get diverted from what they saw was their primary task. This was to use OPV and eradicate the poliovirus from the handful of countries where it was endemic, primarily India, Pakistan, Nigeria and Afghanistan. Their aim was to persuade governments to organise mass immunisation campaigns with OPV over and over again for as many times as was necessary for wild poliovirus to be stamped out. With the repeated deadlines for eradication having slipped by, the polio programme's leadership was fixed on a single goal—to eradicate wild poliovirus as quickly as possible, declare victory and leave. This was regardless of how messy the victory might be in terms of cases of paralytic polio caused by the vaccine virus, or the possible long-term dangers posed by the vaccine virus.

Financially as well, with donors growing weary about the repeated missed deadlines for eradication, a switching to the more expensive inactivated vaccine would have increased the cost of the programme several fold. There was no guarantee that either the countries with endemic polio, or donors would be willing to meet the additional cost. In 2009 a group of outside experts were tasked with producing a position paper on vaccination. Even then the WHO insisted that it should make a 'clear affirmation of eradication of wild polioviruses as the priority, and therefore OPV should be used with the highest possible coverage rates.'[14]

But the weight of epidemiological evidence indicating dangers posed by viruses descended from the oral polio vaccine, and the voices of other WHO expert groups such as SAGE, eventually brought about a formal change in the GPEI's goals in 2012. The polio eradication campaign's plan became not merely wild poliovirus, but also all vaccine-related poliovirus. In what can be seen as a vindication of Jonas Salk's long held views, IPV was to be introduced in stages. Once wild poliovirus had been eradicated, the remaining two components of the oral polio vaccine would be removed from use and only IPV was to be used.

Given the possible persistence of vaccine-derived viruses, current plans call for countries to continue to use IPV for at least a decade after wild poliovirus disappears. This means vaccinating children with a more expensive vaccine for at least a decade after the wild poliovirus is eradicated to protect against a new form of poliovirus caused by the oral polio vaccine. That's not something any of the countries of the world bargained for in 1988 when they voted at the World Health Assembly to eradicate polio.

10

INDIA

A LONG DIRTY WAR

The sprawling, teeming plains of northern India have been the key to the conquest of the subcontinent. It is on this terrain that kings and princes, adventurers and pretenders and an assorted collection of invaders have fought through the centuries to establish kingdoms and empires. It is also in this densely populated land, nurtured by the waters of the Ganges, that the most wrenching battles against pathogens have been fought. Two great global disease eradication campaigns, against smallpox and against polio, came close to collapse here before stumbling to eventual victory.

The viruses were different, the diseases were different, the vaccines were different, and the techniques the two campaigns used were different. But both global efforts faced difficulties in India they would not face elsewhere. These included significant pushback from the government and from Indian medical professionals and a level of popular resistance from sections of the public that it would not encounter elsewhere.

The difficulties the smallpox and polio campaigns faced also shone a harsh and pitiless light on the inadequacies of the Indian public health system, particularly in the country's two poorest, most populous and most poorly governed states, Uttar Pradesh and Bihar. At the same time, the eventual success of the polio and smallpox campaigns also showed that the apparatus of government in even poorly run states was capable of performing at an extremely high level, when pushed to do so.

The experiences of the smallpox campaign foreshadowed the polio programme, so it is useful to glance briefly back to that period. The global campaign to wipe out smallpox was launched in 1958 by the WHO, and India began its effort in 1962. Using vaccine donated by the Soviet Union, over 440 million people were vaccinated between 1962 and 1967. But to everyone's consternation, after this mammoth vaccination effort, there were more cases in 1967 than there had been in 1962. The number of cases in 1967 after five years of vaccination, were the highest they had been in a decade.

Government health staff, the foot soldiers in any eradication campaign, were weary and ready to abandon the effort and the Indian government was ready to throw in the towel. Opinion within the WHO too was divided. WHO staff who were involved in smallpox eradication were convinced they needed to stay the course, others in the organisation felt it was diverting resources away from more pressing health issues. Even the head of the WHO's regional office in New Delhi felt it was a waste of time. 'Dr. Chandra Mani, Director of WHO's South East Asia regional office (SEARO)...was convinced that eradication was impossible. He saw little point in encouraging the Indian government to persist in the futile effort,'[1] wrote DA Henderson, the head of the WHO smallpox unit in Geneva.

Some epidemiologists thought that the smallpox virus had become so entrenched in the population over the centuries that it could never be wiped out. For a start there was the sheer number of people, the crowded conditions in which they lived and the constant, restless movement of hundreds of thousands of men, women and children in search of work. Beyond this the poverty, the insanitary living conditions and a dysfunctional government health system had, it was thought, created a landscape where it would be impossible to stamp out the disease. As the Australian epidemiologist Frank Fenner wrote in a history of the smallpox eradication campaign 'many held the view that because of the population density, or for other ill-defined socio-cultural or epidemiological reasons, the eradication of smallpox in India would ultimately prove impossible.'[2]

The weaknesses of the smallpox campaign between 1962 and 1967 reflected the weakness of governance in many of the Indian states. The machinery of government is a leaky bucket punctured with holes at every level. Orders issued by the central government in New Delhi, or by state governments in their capitals, often evaporate into inaction at the hands of district administrators. A joint Indian government-WHO team travelled the country in 1967 to understand why the smallpox programme had achieved so little in five years. It found that in the districts, 'supervision is poor, morale is low, interest in the programme is fading and vaccine is improperly handled and stored.' They also found that many vaccinators were not doing their job, with some vaccinating an average of less than one person a day. Supervision consisted primarily of checking whether a vaccinator had turned up for work, not on whether any work had been performed.

Nearly five decades later, the global polio campaign would also encounter the same creaky machinery of government in the states of Uttar Pradesh and Bihar. This meant it would struggle to perform tasks as basic as ensuring that every new born child was vaccinated against childhood diseases including polio. One of the arguments against disease eradication has always been that it zeroes in on a single disease and wipes it out, but brings little long-term benefit in the form of improving the basic health services in poor countries. The experience of the poorest states in India bears this out. Between the nearly four decades that separated the end of the smallpox campaign which ended in India and the last case of polio in 2011, two pathogens had been wiped out. But the government machinery delivering health care in India's poorest states had changed little, nor had the overall health of the population.

Both the smallpox and the polio campaigns in India illustrated the often difficult-to-bridge gap between global and national health priorities. Eradicating polio was a global priority. A coalition of powerful global private and public institutions ranging from the WHO to the Gates Foundation and Rotary International had thrown their weight behind this effort and were determined that it would succeed. India had other more pressing priorities to improve in child health. This included increasing the number of children who received their normal childhood immunisations against common diseases like diphtheria and tetanus. (In Uttar Pradesh, only 23 per cent of children under the age of two were estimated to have received all their childhood vaccinations in 2005, while in Bihar it was only 20 per cent.) Except in its final stages, the polio eradication campaign did little to help the overall health system through which routine childhood vaccinations are delivered. In fact, it drained the system by diverting health workers from their normal duties. Vaccination campaigns using the oral polio vaccine were labour intensive. For days and weeks on end, health workers who would otherwise be at primary health centres giving children their childhood shots, or attending to births and newborn children were knocking on doors and dropping vaccine into the mouths of children. And as cases kept see-sawing up and down from 2000, it was not clear whether any end was in sight.

For the WHO and its partners in the polio campaign, there was no doubt that the campaign had to continue till the virus was eradicated. 'We knew we had to do it, and we were going to do it…we weren't going to give up,' said Hamid Jafari, the head of the WHO's polio campaign in India during a crucial period from 2007 to 2012.[3]

But for the Indian government, the calculations were different. Sujatha Rao, the civil servant who headed the Indian Ministry of Health in 2009 and 2010, frequently expressed her frustration to the WHO at the way polio was sucking away resources from other more urgent health needs. 'It completely disrupted the routine immunisation campaign: every three or four months of the year were devoted only to the polio campaign. This meant that those months when the campaign was on, there was no ante-natal care, no routine immunisation done, everything was suspended. This was a huge cost.'[4]

The polio eradication campaign's most anguished and difficult years in India were from 2005 to 2011. This was a period when polio exploded in large, periodic outbreaks in Uttar Pradesh and Bihar, even though the WHO and its partners had thrown the equivalent of the kitchen sink at the virus, with some of the most intensive polio vaccination campaigns the world had seen. Children in parts of western Uttar Pradesh and Bihar were being fed polio drops once a month as opposed to the two times a year that was supposed to be the norm. A new monovalent OPV had been introduced in these states in the hope that at least one of the two poliovirus serotypes could be stamped out. But it was not at all clear that any of this was working. In 2005, after an intensive vaccination campaign with the new monovalent Type 1 vaccine, the number of cases of polio in India had been brought down to a low of fifty-four. This led to optimistic predictions that the disease could be wiped out the following year. But between 2006 and 2008, the numbers had shot up again to nearly 900 cases.

Vaccinators and their supervisors in Uttar Pradesh and Bihar were being stretched to their limits by these repeated campaigns. Some went on strike demanding better payment. Parents were becoming increasingly irritated and suspicious about these repeated knocks on their doors by health workers forcing polio drops on their children.

Could polio actually be wiped out from India? Should the government continue to spend money on eradicating polio, or should it rather use the money to focus on other diseases, officials asked. Was OPV as effective as the WHO claimed it was? All the questions and doubts that had been raised since the 1960s about the right strategy to eradicate polio surfaced again. Should the polio campaign use IPV instead of OPV? Should a combination of the two be tried? Should the polio campaign get involved in strengthening routine childhood immunisation instead of concentrating solely on delivering polio vaccine through house-to-house campaigns? Should improving sanitation and hygiene, be seen as part of the polio eradication mission?

It was not just the government that was sceptical. A group of Indian doctors and epidemiologists also felt that the strategies the WHO was pursuing would lead nowhere. The Indian Academy of Paediatrics, an umbrella organisation for the country's paediatricians, felt that WHO's reliance on OPV alone was unwise, given that efficacy of the vaccine was low in the environmental and social conditions that existed in the heavily populated states of northern India. Some decades earlier in the 1990s, there had been a proposal to start manufacturing IPV in India, but that never got off the ground. However, there remained a strong body of professional opinion that favoured using IPV as well as OPV.

It was in India that the debates over the dangers of the Sabin vaccine and its propensity to provoke paralysis in some recipients, or vaccine associated paralytic poliomyelitis (VAPP) was brought back under the spotlight. The polio programme and the Indian government never publicly talked about OPV's known propensity to cause paralysis, at the rate of roughly one child being paralysed per million doses of vaccine distributed. This rate of paralysis was small, but given the scale of India, where around 150 to 160 million doses were administered at each national immunisation day, as well as the additional doses that children were given during sub national immunisation rounds, several hundred children were developing polio from the vaccine.

Besides, OPV could also revert to a disease-causing state and circulate in communities like the wild poliovirus and cause disease. The WHO and the polio programme justified use of the vaccine on the grounds that this risk needed to be balanced against the benefit of a polio-free world. The Indian government had no interest in discussing publicising these risks of the vaccine because it could lead to claims of compensation from children who were affected by the vaccine (as had happened in the United States). IPV did not have these side effects, and the Indian Academy of Paediatrics urged the Indian government to introduce IPV in addition to the OPV in order to reduce these risks.

It was also in India that a question that ticks like a bomb beneath every global health initiative surfaced again: who was polio eradication a priority for? Was it a priority for India where so many other diseases demanded greater attention? Or was it more of a priority for the wealthy developing countries that had eliminated the disease, but did not want to face the threat of it being reimported from countries where it still circulated? This was a question that public health experts in the West critical of the concept of eradication had raised decades earlier. This argument had more or less disappeared from the discourse in the West, but it re-emerged with new vigour from Indian academics, who found the emphasis on polio questionable. A 'Memorandum on Pulse Polio' submitted to the WHO and UNICEF in New Delhi by a group of academics from Jawaharlal Nehru University in New Delhi claimed that the polio eradication initiative had been thrust on India by the WHO, UNICEF, the US Centers for Disease Control and Rotary. It continued that a, 'disease of lower public health importance in the country has been justified on the grounds of some small saving for developed nations.'[5]

A group of Indian doctors and academics, dubbed the 'dissenters' by the historian William Muraskin, subjected the polio campaign to the kind of critical scrutiny that it was not accustomed to anywhere else in the world. The polio campaign blamed the health authorities in the problem states of UP and Bihar for not implementing immunisation campaigns with sufficient care and rigor. Yet Indian critics wrote 'the failure of the eradication campaign is not because of a lack of proper implementation (as they so often claim) but because of a flawed strategy itself.'[6] Many of these objections were valid, and others less so. But it is to the credit of the polio programme that it persisted, and mobilised the political support it needed from the central and state governments to bulldoze ahead until polio disappeared from India.

Despite often valid criticism of the campaign, the eradication of the poliovirus from India will go down as a magnificent chapter in the history of public health. It was achieved by meticulous implementation of a vaccination programme that reached children in some of the most physically and epidemiologically challenging environments that the polio programme had ever encountered. These ranged from the squalid slums where sewage and drinking water ran together, to remote huts on the flood plains of the Kosi river in Bihar where no health care worker had ever gone before. As we shall see in the following section, nowhere else had the poliovirus been successfully hunted down in conditions that were so challenging.

* * *

Exterminating a virus thousands of times more minuscule than the smallest grain of sand, from a country as large, as poor and as densely populated as India, was never going to be easy. Not least given the country's creaky public health system and often chaotic administration. But the early stages of polio eradication proceeded so smoothly that no one foresaw the morass in which the campaign would find itself in northern India.

India began administering OPV to children as part of routine childhood vaccinations on a small scale in the late 1970s. This was even before the 1988 WHO resolution to eradicate polio. Public health clinics, hospitals and private doctors would include three doses of OPV along with shots against diphtheria, tetanus and whooping cough. This saw a sharp reduction in the estimated number of polio cases in the country, from over 27,000 in 1985, to a little over 3,000 cases in 1995.

This method of administering polio drops to children whenever they happened to come to a clinic, was suitable for reducing the number of cases of polio, but it was not suited to eradicating the virus. For the virus to be eradicated, you needed simultaneous mass immunisation of hundreds of millions of children.

POLIO

With the year 2000 deadline for polio eradication looming, the WHO began to urge countries to introduce such mass immunisation days to stamp out the virus. After pilot campaigns in the states of Kerala, Tamil Nadu and the Delhi capital region, India launched its first nationwide campaign in December 1995. Known in India as Pulse Polio Immunisation, it was the start of a process that would grind on for well over a decade.

The early national immunisation days were festive occasions. Instead of vaccinators going door-to-door, polio drops were distributed at booths, decorated by buntings and posters, often manned by Rotarians. Vans with loudspeakers and music would drive by urging parents to give their children polio drops. 'The festive atmosphere at the booths was important, and Rotary played a big role in that. Putting up bunting, providing little giveaways for the children like rubber or plastic balls. One time we gave away whistles all over the country,' Deepak Kapur, the head of Rotary's polio efforts in India recalled.[7] A UNICEF report noted that the early immunisation days, 'enjoyed enormous popularity as a people's programme, unleashing a tremendous spirit of volunteerism... large numbers of volunteers including teachers, students, religious leaders, medical practitioners, housewives, community leaders came forward...Throughout the country, school children took to the streets in droves to raise awareness of National Immunisation Day. Villagers pedalled loudspeakers around while rows of young people marched to the rhythmic beat of drums, publicizing the day with much fanfare and colour.'[8] Had Albert Sabin been alive, he would have looked on approvingly. This was how he had intended his vaccine to be used: in large, community-driven immunisation drives, with eager parents and excited children waiting to get their polio drops.

The early immunisation rounds were successful: nearly 90 million children were given polio drops in December 1995, in the largest such exercise the world had seen to date. The Sabin vaccine worked its magic, and by 2000, the poliovirus appeared to have retreated from most of the country to the western districts of Uttar Pradesh and Bihar, with a few cases spilling over into the neighbouring states of West Bengal to the east, and Delhi and Punjab to the west. The WHO was confident that even though the 2000 target had been missed, polio could be wiped out by 2001. A few more high-quality immunisation campaigns offered 'the promise that this region will interrupt wild poliovirus transmission in the next six to twelve months' the WHO predicted.[9]

The poliovirus however fought back from its place of refuge in the poorest districts of the two of the poorest states of the country, Uttar Pradesh and Bihar. Here the the lack of health care services, poor hygiene and sanitation provided it shelter to multiply and spread for more than a decade after the initial predictions that India would be polio-free by 2001.

As the campaign ground on, the enthusiasm that surrounded the annual immunisation drives in the 1990s also evaporated. Polio immunisation also gradually changed from being volunteer driven to being run by the government health services. As the number of immunisation days increased it was no longer possible for volunteers to participate in what had become a full-time job.

The method of delivering vaccines became more intensive. In addition to 'booth days' when parents would bring their children to vaccination booths and stalls, vaccinators would also go house-to-house in pursuit of the poliovirus, knocking on every door, and vaccinating every child they could find. And they would do this not just twice a year, but on an almost monthly basis. As the campaign progressed, it was not just one team that was involved, but two teams: an A team that would vaccinate on one day, and a B team that would follow up a day or two later to knock on doors where children had not been vaccinated by the A team.

The government health system began to slowly buckle under the stress of repeated vaccination campaigns, held on a scale that existed in no other country.

On immunisation days more than 2 million vaccinators would collect carrier bags of polio vaccine from government health centres, and begin several days of work. This would see them knocking on over 200 million homes across the country (each vaccinator was expected to visit an average of 100 homes) and squeeze polio drops into the mouths of around 160 to 170 million children under five years old.

Each immunisation day would be preceded by weeks of preparation. Vaccine supplies would have to be ordered well in advance and delivered to distribution centres across the subcontinent. Jeeps and vans and buses had to be requisitioned from government departments to carry the vaccines to often remote government clinics and health centres where they would be stored in freezers until the day of the campaign. Community health workers and the staff of government primary health centres and clinics would be drafted in as vaccinators. Detailed rosters would be drawn up of vaccinators and their routes. The lanes and alleyways they would take, and the doors they would knock on were mapped out in advance. The vaccinators would mark each door with a set of symbols: P (indicating that children had already been vaccinated), X (indicating the door was locked and the house needed to be revisited), XR (indicating the family had refused vaccination). A day or two later, a follow-up team of vaccinators would visit to knock on the doors with X on them to persuade parents to get their children immunised. Supervisors would collect data on the number of children immunised and the number of children missed. They would pass this up the hierarchy until it reached the offices of the National Polio Surveillance Programme in New Delhi, the organisation that the WHO and the Indian government had set up to run the polio eradication campaign.

Each immunisation day would be preceded by a publicity campaign of posters and radio and television advertisements. India's biggest film star, Amitabh Bachchan, who occupied an almost god-like status among his millions of fans was drafted in producing television spots urging parents to vaccinate their children. The army of vaccinators was preceded by a slightly smaller army of 'community mobilisers', or village level communicators, normally women from the area, who would knock on doors and with the help of brightly coloured booklets explain to parents how important it was to get their children vaccinated against polio. These community mobilisers were in turn supervised by a hierarchy of supervisors.

In theory, these immunisation days should have seen polio eliminated from India after a few years. OPV was less effective in India and other tropical countries than it was in more temperate climes. Since it was least effective in the populous states of Uttar Pradesh and Bihar, these immunisation rounds were held as often as once every two months in certain districts.

Nowhere else in the world had the polio vaccine been used with such intensity. Or with such little effect. 'There were figures showing that children getting ten doses, twelve doses of OPV were still getting polio', recalled Jacob John.[10] A study was carried out by Nicholas Grassly, an epidemiologist at Imperial College in London. It found that a single dose of trivalent OPV only offered 9 per cent protection against Type 1 poliovirus (the most aggressive poliovirus and the strain that was causing most outbreaks against in UP and Bihar during 2000–2005).[11] That implied that even after fifteen doses, there was still a 10 per cent chance that a child could be infected with polio.

Eradication campaigns are extremely intensive, but they are meant to be quick, time-bound activities. A country puts in an intense effort for a short period of time and knocks out a disease forever: that is the logic of eradication. When the intense effort has to carry on month after month, and year after year with success uncertain, diverting resources from other urgent health needs, that is when governments and the public begin to push back, as happened in India.

It also led to what came to be described as 'campaign fatigue' on the part of vaccinators who knocked on the same doors repeatedly, repeated exactly the same script to reluctant parents and put up with increasing hostility from them.

The low efficacy of the vaccine to an extent reflected the wretched state of health and public administration in the two states where the poliovirus managed to entrench itself.

As the nineteenth-century German physician Rudolf Virchow—the founder of social medicine—would have put it, the health of a people is a reflection of the society they live in. Uttar Pradesh and Bihar are two of the most populous and most underdeveloped states in the country. Both have the highest rates of infant mortality in the country: seventy-one out of every 1,000 children in Uttar Pradesh die before they see their first birthday, as do sixty out of every 1,000 children in Bihar. By comparison, in Kerala, India's most advanced state in terms of social and economic indicators, fifteen out of every 1,000 children died before the age of one. The high infant mortality rate in these states is in turn a reflection of the poverty of health services and poor sanitation. Diarrhoea is a major killer of children in their first year of birth and three quarters of children in the state of Uttar Pradesh are born at home in unhygienic conditions. Less than a quarter of mothers receive antenatal care from doctors. At the time of the campaign, nearly 71 per cent of all children in both these states under the age of three were believed to have iron deficiency anaemia. And only 23 per cent of children under the age of two had received all their routine childhood vaccinations: a figure that was to have an impact on the fate of the polio eradication campaign. In Bihar, only 20 per cent of children were estimated to have received their regular childhood vaccinations. This combination of high rates of diarrhoeal disease, crowded, unsanitary living conditions and poor nutrition, all served to reduce the effectiveness of the vaccine.

Both states also had a reputation for being among the worst-administered in the country, and the fate of the polio campaign was often caught in the political instability that often swept them. The 2000–2003 period in Uttar Pradesh, when cases of polio exploded from around 250 cases to 1242 in 2002, was also a period of political instability. The party ruling the state, the Bharatiya Janata Party, witnessed a variety of party leaders vying to lead the government. Bihar was led by a charismatic, but notoriously corrupt populist leader, Lalu Prasad Yadav. In 2004, the *Economist* magazine famously described the state as a 'byword for the worst of India, of widespread and inescapable poverty, of corrupt politicians indistinguishable from the mafia dons they patronise.'[12] Poor administration and governance in turn meant that the poor did not have access to vaccines and other health care: the polio vaccine was simply not reaching them.

The poverty, maladministration and social divisions in these states as well as the poverty and poor health created a cocktail of conditions that tested the polio eradication campaign to its limits. The first warning came in 2002, when the number of polio cases in India exploded from 250 the previous year to 1600. This was over 80 per cent of the cases recorded globally that year. And the bulk of these cases in turn were clustered among Muslims in western Uttar Pradesh. And poor Muslims were hit the hardest.

Viruses often find sanctuary among those who live on the margins of society, or those who feel excluded from the rest of society. Riots between Hindus and Muslims, particularly in the late 1980s and early 1990s had led to a ghettoisation of poor Muslims, and a suspicion among Muslims of the state government. 'The government generally does not want to develop these areas. They know they don't get votes from these areas, so they will only develop the areas from which they get the votes,' was a typical comment from a Muslim in the town of Aligarh in western Uttar Pradesh.[13] The conditions in the areas they lived and where the poliovirus propagated were wretched. 'Huge loads of unattended solid waste chokes up sewers, pollutes water pipes, spills over open drains permeating the air with a foul, putrid stench. Human and animal faeces, wet ones, dried ones line every alleyway,'[14] was how one UNICEF report described conditions in a poor part of Meerut city in Uttar Pradesh.

Polio spread in these communities because few of them immunised their children regularly, a knock-on effect from the close to non-existent public health services. A study commissioned by UNICEF recorded the following observations about the government health services. 'The nurse scolds us saying why do you produce so many children, and the doctors do not bother about those who do not have money,' said one Muslim respondent. This reflected the belief in the community that the government health services were not there to serve them.

The polio programme's response to the rise in polio cases among Muslims was to vaccinate children in these communities as often as possible. The repeated vaccination campaigns in turn stoked suspicions. Why was a government that provided little or no health services suddenly interested in repeatedly providing free vaccination for a disease that was not as common as more serious causes of death and illness among children? 'Why is this polio medicine being given? Everybody will be suspicious. If you give only one curative, then people will definitely suspect,' an elderly Muslim woman was quoted as saying in a focus group discussion carried out for a study commissioned by the WHO and UNICEF. The increasing frequency of vaccination campaigns led many to come to the entirely reasonable conclusion that the vaccine was not every effective. 'Our nephew also has polio. He has been given the vaccine. How did he manage to get the disease despite taking the medicine?' commented a 30-year-old Muslim woman from Ghaziabad in western Uttar Pradesh.[15] 'Even if we give the vaccine, our children are liable to get polio,' commented another survey respondent.

Comments such as these on the effectiveness of the polio vaccine, were described as arising from ignorance and the poor educational level of the respondents. Elaborate communication campaigns were devised by UNICEF to counter what were seen as misperceptions on the part of poor, simple people. But these were entirely rational questions, and were the same ones being asked at the highest levels of the polio campaign in Geneva. Alternate strategies such as using monovalent vaccines, and possibly introducing IPV were being considered to counter the low efficacy of OPV.

In the hierarchy of global power and knowledge, questions asked by those at the top of the hierarchy are treated in a very different way to the same questions being asked at the bottom of the global hierarchy. Beyond this there are the questions that are not based on fact, but if not addressed properly can cause significant problems of their own. Among the Muslim community, rumours were rife that the polio vaccine was intended to sterilise Muslims and reduce their population. This belief also spread in Nigeria around the same period of time, and would be echoed in Pakistan at a slightly later period. In the Muslim areas of northern Nigeria local preachers argued that sterilising Muslims was part of the West's revenge for the 9/11 attacks on the United States. In India, suspicion about the vaccine was also a reflection of the state of the government health services. The only other free health intervention that was delivered to people's doors was contraception. And it was the same government health workers who delivered contraception, who were now bringing oral polio vaccine to people's doors.

The wretched conditions in the slums where poorer Muslims lived, also contributed to anger and outrage. Local leaders began using polio as a bargaining chip to force the local government to improve sanitation and infrastructure. The frustration of ordinary people would erupt when polio vaccinators, the only representative of the government machinery they ever saw, knocked on their doors. 'Don't talk about polio, my children are all under five, just look at my squalid conditions,' raged a middle-aged woman, pulling Subaida Khatoon a Muslim CMC (a community level mobiliser for the polio campaign) into her makeshift kitchen. She pointed to the sink overflowing with oily, brownish water congealing into mud.'[16]

Many, quite rightly, equated the lack of basic sanitation and hygiene as the reason the poliovirus continued to transmit in their communities, even though their children had often been vaccinated multiple times. One researcher asked a poor labourer in Aligarh for his views on why polio spread, and got this response: 'The filth...the government does not stop it. If only the filth could be finished off.'[17]

The questions poor Muslims in western Uttar Pradesh raised, were responses to the contradictory nature of disease eradication. The aim of disease eradication was to eradicate a pathogen, in this case the poliovirus. It was not to improve the general health of the population by improving sanitation. Nor was it reducing maternal mortality, or providing a better chance of a child surviving its first year of life by providing access to childhood immunisation, or having qualified birth attendants to childbirth. The logic of eradication was to bypass all these other barriers to better health and zero in on a single pathogen. For those at the receiving end, this strategy made little sense, especially since the pathogen in question was not the most serious threat to children's health.

The polio campaign described those who questioned the polio campaign and did not want their children to have multiple doses of polio vaccine as 'resistors' suffering from 'misperceptions'. Their doors were marked with XR, and elaborate communication plans were created by UNICEF, CORE, a group of US NGOs, and Rotary to persuade them to get their children immunised as often as was necessary.

Any account of the polio programme in India has to take note of the gigantic communication effort that went into persuading people in Uttar Pradesh and Bihar to get their children immunised against polio. The bedrock of the communication effort was the Social Mobilisation Network (SMNet). This network was based on women (and a few men) from local communities. They would be trained to go house-to-house, meet with families, build relationships with them, and persuade them that the polio vaccine was safe and that they needed to get their children immunised as often as possible.

India has had a history of programmes to introduce community level village workers, none of which have worked particularly well. UNICEF and its polio partners demonstrated through meticulous planning, training and implementation of how such an army of community level workers should function. Besides their ability to talk to local families, these women were also taught to be record keepers. They had to conduct surveys of how many children under the age of five (the target group of polio vaccination) each household had, have meetings with 'resistant families' until they were 'converted'. They also had to track newborn children so they could get a quick initial dose of polio. They were trained to use management tools such as resource maps, monthly work plans and microplans mapping the households in the areas they worked in.

Since this network was initially set up to focus on the Muslim community, and the community workers were for the most part Muslim women, they were also trained to talk about vaccination in a religious context. They talked about the need to protect children who are a gift from Allah, to keep the mind and body free from disease and, how it was important to prevent diseases.[18]

In addition to these community-level workers, high profile Muslim imams were also drafted into the polio campaign to use their Friday sermons to urge worshippers to get their children vaccinated. A key figure in this was the head of a prominent mosque in Lucknow in Uttar Pradesh, Khalid Rashid Firangi Mahali. Mahali helped the polio campaign find a leading Muslim scholar in every district to form a committee that would spread messages in support of polio immunisation. This intensive campaign for the polio vaccination eventually wore down the resistance of the resistors, and vaccination rates in the Muslim community increased.

While poor Muslims refused vaccination even though it was being brought to them, there were other poor non-Muslims who were not reached by polio vaccinators, or by any health service for that matter. This was because poverty had pushed them to the outer fringes of society, beyond the reach of the health system. Many were wretchedly poor migrant workers, making their way across the Gangetic plain to find work on construction sites and brick kilns. There they would live in small colonies, in flimsy, makeshift shelters, with no clean water and sanitation. While the adults worked making bricks, breaking stone, the children ran around, often malnourished, underweight and prey to every common infection. Some belonged to traditional nomadic groups, living in makeshift huts and shelters wherever they decided to stop: beside railway stations, near marketplaces or on the edges of existing slums. These nomadic families had little contact with more established local populations who tended to view them with suspicion and would look down upon them.

It is one of the great triumphs of the polio campaign, that polio vaccinators managed to reach these families, who had been had been forgotten, ignored and looked down upon throughout the country's history.

To discover who these communities were, where they lived and how
best to reach them, the WHO and UNICEF performed one of the most
detailed mapping exercises that had ever been conducted of these marginal communities. UNICEF recruited a network of over 20,000 inform-
ers such as local shopkeepers, and owners of brick kilns, or even local
residents who would provide information whenever new families of
migrants arrived in the neighbourhood. Based on information from this
network of informants around 40,000 sites where migrant populations
tended to live were mapped out. Over 20,000 migrant families who
travelled as far as Mumbai in the west and West Bengal in the east were
identified. Community workers were hired to contact these families, win
their support and get their children immunised against polio. Once identified the WHO included them in their micro plans, or detailed household and community maps, and vaccinators were dispatched.

Mobile teams were formed to vaccinate children of migrant workers
as they travelled. Vaccinators would jump onto trains and walk down
the carriages, putting drops into the mouths of children they thought
would be five years or under. Teams of vaccinators would wander
through railway stations and bus terminals and other transit points to
vaccinate children. Other vaccination teams would be stationed on the
busy land border between India and Nepal to try to keep the virus
from crossing borders. At one stage eighty-one vaccination posts were
set up all along the border.

Perhaps the remotest and most challenging terrain on which the
poliovirus was pursued in India was along the flood plains of the Kosi
river in northern Bihar, and its tributaries the Kamala and the Kareh.
This was an area that was inaccessible for three to five months of the
year, when the river waters would overflow onto the surrounding
plains. There were few bridges and roads, and the only way to reach
isolated communities was by boat, by motorcycle or on foot. Once
again, the WHO and UNICEF, backed by the district administration
began to map and enumerate communities that no one had paid any
attention to before. Since travel was difficult, shelters were set up where
vaccinators and supervisors could spend up to ten days at a time.

No other health programme in India had put in such a meticulously planned and executed campaign to reach the often invisible children in the poorest of the country's poor families. By the end of 2009, surveys indicated that the polio campaign had succeeded in reaching 97 per cent of children even in remote field huts in the Kosi river basin. In Uttar Pradesh, 96 per cent of children in migrant populations had been reached during immunisation campaigns.

With these high levels of vaccination, the poliovirus was getting fewer and fewer opportunities to replicate and it was only a matter of time before it would disappear from India. 'We weren't going to give up, and we knew at some point as we were getting more and more children vaccinated, and missing fewer and fewer children, there would be a tipping point when we would succeed,' observed Hamid Jafari, the WHO's head of the polio campaign in India during this period.[19] But before the last case of polio in India was recorded in early 2011, the polio campaign would have to survive two explosions—one epidemiological, and the other political.

11

TWO CRISES AND A FINAL VICTORY

A quiet, leafy bungalow on the outskirts of the town of Vellore in the southern Indian state of Tamil Nadu, has an unusual detail. Near the front door is a hexagonal porthole shaped window with a pattern of thin, white-painted metal bars behind the glass. I paid little attention to the window when I entered the house. It was only as I left that the owner asked me to look closely at it. The metal bars are arranged in the shape of ten interlocking equilateral triangles. 'That is the shape of a poliovirus, and if you stand back a bit, you can see it stand out in three dimensions,' Jacob John tells me.

The poliovirus-shaped window bars reflect a life that has been spent trying to exterminate the poliovirus. John, a slim, active man in his eighties, can well claim to be India's foremost expert on both the disease and the virus. In the late 1960s he ran one of the first studies to understand how many cases of polio there might be in India.

Those early studies were the beginning of a professional career devoted to understanding and studying polio. This career would lead him to sit on World Health Organisation committees, rub shoulders with Albert Sabin and Jonas Salk, conduct vaccine trials in India, and also chair the main expert group advising the polio group in India. But despite this, Jacob John has always been a maverick in the world of polio and has consistently questioned one of the fundamental articles of faith of the polio campaign. Was the Sabin oral polio vaccine (OPV), the best tool to use to eradicate polio?

John had used OPV in small trials in Vellore in the late 1960s, but found a significant number of children falling ill with polio despite receiving the three doses of vaccine recommended at the time. Clearly it was not as effective in tropical conditions as Sabin and the WHO thought it would be. John's confidence in the vaccine was further diminished in 1982 by a WHO study that showed that the oral polio vaccine was paralysing children at the rate of roughly one child (or a close contact of a child who had been vaccinated) for every two million doses of vaccine that was administered. Despite this, the authors of the study concluded that the oral polio vaccine was 'one of the safest vaccines in use.'[1]

John was troubled by this description of the oral vaccine as being safe. 'This vaccine can cause paralysis, it can cause hospitalisation. There are only two vaccines that I consider to be unsafe: one is the old rabies vaccine (based on infected neural tissue) and the other is the oral polio vaccine.'[2] John felt the only reason the WHO study had described OPV as a safe vaccine was because of Sabin's influence. 'Albert Sabin was a member of the committee that did the study. The wording about it being one of the safest vaccines was his wording. If they had really wanted to look at the vaccine independently, they should not have included him in the committee.'[3] John began a long campaign against the use of OPV, and in favour of the Salk IPV as a better tool to wipe out polio. John was chair of the India Expert Advisory Group on polio eradication(IEAG)—the body that advised the polio campaign and the Indian government on the strategies to be followed to achieve eradication. It is perhaps one of the ironies of polio eradication in India that in that role he presided over one of the most intensive uses of OPV in Bihar and Uttar Pradesh the world had seen to date. He took decisions that were successful in the end, but also raised their own ethical concerns.

Crucial decisions were taken between 2004 and 2009 to introduce new monovalent forms of OPV that were more effective than the traditional trivalent vaccine. The aim was also to concentrate on first eliminating Type 1 poliovirus, which had caused all the big explosions in India to date and spread more aggressively than Type 3.

The new monovalent Type 1 OPV at first had an almost magical effect in reducing the amount of Type 1 poliovirus transmitting in northern India. The number of polio cases caused by the virus fell sharply, and the WHO's polio epidemiologists were cheered by the fact that all these cases seemed to be coming from just two genetic clusters of virus. The greater the genetic diversity of a virus (or any living organism) the harder it is to stamp out. The less the genetic diversity, the more vulnerable it is to extinction. It also looked as though the Type 3 virus, which spreads less easily than Type 1 was about to disappear: only three cases were recorded in 2005, all from Bihar. There was optimism that within a year, polio could be stamped out from India.

But polioviruses are living organisms that have survived over hundreds of thousands of years by learning to survive, by exploiting any opportunity to find new hosts and multiply. And in 2006, the Type 1 virus found an escape route in the town of Moradabad in western Uttar Pradesh. The pockets of the town and surrounding district where poorer Muslim families lived had been untouched by the bi-monthly vaccination campaigns. They were suspicious of the vaccines and as a result over the years a large number of children had been left either unimmunised or under-immunised. Only about 10 per cent of households had skipped or missed out on polio vaccines. But given the density of population this still meant tens of thousands of children living in conditions that favoured polio transmission: crowded living conditions, and poor sanitation. This was enough for the virus to explode and spread not merely within Uttar Pradesh and Bihar, but to twelve other states.

This explosion of cases a year after the polio eradication campaign had confidently predicted that with the new monovalent vaccine, the Type 1 virus was on the verge of disappearing, predictably raised questions about the WHO's strategies and overall competence. It also increased pressure on the Indian government to answer for the rise in cases. Parliamentarians began to raise questions about the effectiveness of the vaccine, and the government's strategy.

'Will the Minister for Health and Family Welfare be pleased to state whether despite the efforts made by the Government of India under the polio eradication programme, there has been an increase in the number of polio cases during the current year?' This was one typical question asked in May 2006, as polio cases began to rise. The ministerial response typically pushed responsibility to the WHO and stated that the government was only following strategies that the India Expert Advisory Group (IEAG) had suggested.

The only solution, as John the chair of the IEAG and the WHO both saw it, was to keep hammering away at the Type 1 virus with the monovalent OPV. An essential element of this was trying to reach children in communities that were being missed by polio vaccinators. The epidemiology of polio in India had shown a pattern of explosive outbreaks of Type 1 polio every four years or so. There had been a big explosion in 1998, another one in 2002 and now the same thing had happened in 2006. 'I knew that Type 1 came with a predictable regularity, and I predicted the next outbreak would be in 2010, and it was important to prevent that,' John recalled.

But this strategy of focusing on the Type 1 virus left an immunity gap: children were well protected against Type 1, but had no protection against Type 3 virus. A cohort of several million children had been left completely vulnerable to Type 3 virus. Given the poliovirus's survival instincts, it was inevitable that this gap would be found and exploited by the virus.

The Shravani Mela in Bihar, is an annual a festival to celebrate the arrival of the monsoon rains in July–August. Hundreds of thousands of people, including children, travel on a 100km pilgrimage from the Ganges. It was just the opportunity the poliovirus needed. The large numbers of people camping in shelters with no sanitation allowed the virus to hop from person to person easily. Every day, the walking pilgrims would drop the virus off at new places along the route, allowing it to infect new groups of people. Inevitably, in 2007 an outbreak of Type 3 polio occurred among pilgrims. It spread all over Uttar Pradesh, Bihar and to thirteen other states paralysing over 1,000 children before it was brought under control.

The polio programme was now struggling to control two epidemics: a Type 1 epidemic that had begun in 2006, and a Type 3 epidemic. Despite five years of hammering away at the poliovirus with round after round of vaccination, polio in India appeared to be going back to where it was in the 1990s.

The WHO's credibility was in tatters. Even among the polio campaign partners, there was dismay. 'We all lost heart constantly,' recalled Deepak Kapur of Rotary. 'We were constantly wondering what was happening. We used to ring up Jacob John and ask him what was happening. He would say keep plugging away with the monovalent Type 1.'[4]

Polio epidemiologists tend to look at disease outbreaks through a different lens than those outside the world of epidemiology do. So, while the government and the public experienced an explosion of polio cases, those within the world of polio saw something else. While Type 3 cases were exploding, John and the WHO polio team were taking heart from the rapidly falling number of Type 1 cases. Type 3 could be taken care off after Type 1 was stamped out.

While this strategy may have made sense epidemiologically it was ethically suspect. The neglect of Type 3 and the focus on Type 1 had led to a manmade, or iatrogenic epidemic of over 1,000 cases of Type 3, as several influential voices pointed out. R K Agarwal, the then president of the Indian Academy of Pediatrics, wrote in 2008 that while technically the decision to focus on Type 1 could be justified, 'on ethical grounds it raises serious concerns. The epidemiology of Type 1 and Type 3 may have stark differences, but at a host level the end results are the same. The paralysis caused by Type 3 is no less severe than the one caused by other types.' Agarwal was in no doubt that the WHO's (or to be more precise the India Expert Advisory Group's) tactics were to blame for these several hundred cases of paralysis. 'WHO has quite deliberately taken the risk of letting Type 3 run loose, especially in highly endemic districts of UP and Bihar...as a result the entire 0–5 population was susceptible to infection... It would not be inappropriate to term the recent epidemic of Type 3 as iatrogenic.'[5]

It was not only experts from outside the polio programme who were dismayed by the use of a vaccination strategy that allowed this outbreak to occur. There was unhappiness among polio experts at the US CDC, perhaps the WHO's closest partner on technical strategy. 'We created a manmade outbreak...I was very upset about that,' recalled Steve Cochi, one of the US CDC's most experienced polio experts, and a member of the India Expert Advisory Group. 'WHO kept using the Type 1 monovalent instead of alternating the use of Type 1 and Type 3... the result was a ping pong effect, with reduced population immunity to Type 3.... It was almost a thousand cases of Type 3 that would not have otherwise happened... Those are the days I would like to forget.'[6]

The Type 3 virus eventually died out in 2009, as did the Type 1 virus in early 2011, but the road was messy and ethically dubious. John, when he looks back on that period, is still convinced that there was little option but to hit away relentlessly at the more aggressive Type 1 if polio was to be eradicated. 'We had a carefully crafted strategy to end polio in India and though the Type 3 attacks were unexpected, they were not as alarming as Type 1. We needed to keep our nerve: cool nerves and clear thinking were necessary.'[7]

Though the eruption of Type 3 cases was an ethically fraught issue, for John, the real ethical issue was the polio campaign's use of OPV. A far safer and more effective alternative existed in the form of IPV. In the mid 1980s John had run a trial in Vellore of the vaccine, and found that two doses of IPV protected children against paralysis. 'Two doses produced 100 per cent sero-conversion, if you have the first dose at fourteen weeks and the second dose at least two months later,' he recalled. This level of protection was far superior to the oral polio vaccine, where even three doses only offered 70 per cent protection.

But since the Salk vaccine had been ruled out by the WHO and the Indian government, as John saw it, the only way to achieve eradication was to use the oral polio vaccine in the most efficient way possible. This meant targeting the most aggressively spreading type of poliovirus, Type 1, first. 'I always say there are three Es involved: ethics, economics and epidemiology. I went for the epidemiology, and ethical issues cropped up periodically, but people couldn't decide how they were to change the vaccine (to IPV) for the sake of ethics.'

* * *

The manmade explosion of Type 3 polio cases would paralyse over 1,200 children during 2007 and 2008 and trigger a political explosion at the November 2009 meeting of the India Expert Advisory Group. The polio eradication campaign was given a clear indication that the Indian government was not going to continue indefinitely with a programme that seemed to have no end in sight.

Sujatha Rao, a former head of the Indian AIDS control programme, had recently been appointed the Health Secretary, or senior most civil servant, in the Indian Ministry of Health in the second half of 2009. She chaired the November IEAG meeting along with John. Seen from her vantage point in the Ministry of Health—with all the other urgent health issues that needed to be dealt with—the resource-hungry polio campaign was becoming a drag. The almost monthly vaccination campaigns in Bihar and Uttar Pradesh, as well as the two national immunisation days were putting a stress on the government health system that could not be maintained for ever. 'At that first meeting, I asked how long can we continue with this polio campaign? Because of the campaign I am not unable to continue with the unfinished agenda of increasing the rate of routine immunisation, nor could I take the step of introducing new vaccines. We had other reasons that children died, so there had to be some finality to it. Because Bihar had polio cases, the rest of the country could not be held to ransom, and we could not keep holding our breath for polio to end.'[8]

By November 2009, there was no doubt that India was fatigued by a polio eradication campaign that involved delivering polio drops house-to-house, month after month. 'India was getting tired. There was a strike by health workers saying we will not do these endless campaigns. The burdens from other diseases were getting larger, our health agendas were complex, and we needed to focus on other things. It was not possible to continue with these monthly and bi-monthly campaigns for ever,' she recalled.

Polio vaccinators were regular field workers in the public health system, and included the midwives who were responsible for antenatal care. 'Three months of their work was taken away for polio campaigns. This meant that during those months, no antenatal care was done, no routine immunisation was done, this was a huge cost.' The draining away of resources from routine immunisation and primary health care was having an impact on children's health. 'Measles, which accounted for 6 per cent of child mortality was being neglected, diphtheria was reappearing in certain parts… You had over 90 per cent coverage in polio campaigns, but only 60 per cent for routine immunisation. Why was there this disparity?'

Rao's questions to the polio campaign were backed by Jaya Prakash Muliyil, an epidemiologist and professor of community medicine from Christian Medical College, Vellore, who Sujatha Rao had brought onto the IEAG. Muliyil strongly argued for a greater focus on strengthening routine immunisation, rather than persisting with an unsustainable method of delivering vaccines door-to-door, even if this meant polio eradication took longer to achieve. 'I said you have to strengthen primary vaccination… we need to create a sustainable mode of delivery.'[9]

This might well mean that eradication would take longer to achieve, but Muliyil argued that these timelines were man-made. The important thing was to ensure that the methods used were sustainable. Muliyil also argued that without improving sanitation and hygiene and improving water conditions it would be difficult to definitively demonstrate that the virus had actually disappeared.

IEAG meetings had never been places where the basic premises of polio eradication were questioned. The Director of the WHO polio programme in Geneva, Bruce Aylward, an expert from the US CDC, three or four Indian experts, a senior official from the Indian Ministry of Health, and representatives from Rotary and UNICEF would meet twice a year in New Delhi. With them would be international donors such as USAID and DFID to look at the number of cases of polio and tell the Indian government how many rounds of vaccination should be conducted over the next couple of months. The agenda was usually structured around three or four questions, including an assessment of where the campaign was, the risks that lay are ahead, and what the central and state governments should be doing to implement vaccination campaigns better. The IEAG would meet for two days, make its recommendations, and the same process would be repeated six months later. The recommendations invariably included a note of congratulation on the progress that had been achieved so far, and messages urging the government not to let up on its efforts.

This was the first time the basic premises of the polio campaign had been questioned. Rao, had brought in a critical outsider's view to the polio campaign in India, and raised the questions that have always haunted single disease eradication programmes. Would the health of children be better served by hammering away at a single virus, or by spreading efforts more broadly? What was the role of sanitation and hygiene in protecting children from polio as well as other diseases? Should this also be a focus of the polio campaign?

From the perspective of the global polio eradication initiative, such questions spelt disaster. The GPEI was an organisation that had been created with a single objective: to stamp out the poliovirus using OPV in intensive house-to-house campaigns. Any deviation from this objective was simply not possible. More than US$17 billion had been spent over more than three decades, and if the campaign was to be wound up, the reputation of all future global health programmes would be at stake. At a personal level as well, all the WHO staff on the polio eradication campaign from Bruce Aylward downward, were completely committed to achieving eradication. In some cases they had spent more than a decade of their lives trying to stamp out the poliovirus.

At the November meeting, Bruce Aylward in particular argued forcefully for the Indian government to stay the course, defending the strategies that the polio campaign had used. John, who was not often on the same side as the WHO, also argued that the Indian government had undertaken a commitment to eradicate polio and that it could not back away.

According to Rao, the Indian government at the time had no intention of pulling out of the polio eradication effort. 'The question of pulling out was never there. Politically it (the polio eradication campaign) gave excellent optics, and political commitment was very strong.' But at the same time, the government wanted to make it clear that its patience was not endless, and that there was a real cost to the programme dragging on in terms of missed opportunities in other areas of health care.

After the IEAG meeting, there was a tacit agreement that India would keep the polio campaign going for another two years, by which time the job had to be done. Bill Gates, the big weapon that the polio campaign wheeled out whenever governments appeared to be flagging made a trip to India and argued that India was at the finishing post and should not flag. 'He kept saying it will be eradicated in two years, and you are at the last mile,' Sujatha Rao recalled.

But this pushback from the government was having an effect, at least at the surface level, on the polio campaign's strategies. A bivalent form of OPV that combined both Type 1 and Type 3 was introduced in 2010 and was probably instrumental in helping to stamp out polio by 2011. At the same time, instead of merely pumping endless rounds of vaccine, the Indian government and the WHO decided to also try to improve drinking water quality through chlorination. On top of this they provided zinc supplementation and oral rehydration salts to prevent diarrhoea, and also worked to use the polio programme's significant ability to reach populations outside the reach of normal health services to strengthen routine childhood immunisation. This was tried in 107 blocks (a block is a sub-unit of a district) in Uttar Pradesh and Bihar that were believed to be at high risk of polio outbreaks.

The Indian government described this strategy by saying, 'The 107 Block Plan…expands the scope of our polio eradication programme beyond delivering OPV vaccination. It will enable us to deliver a more complete package of services like routine immunisation services and improved health and sanitation services so that children can only not only be free of polio, but also have a healthy childhood.'[10]

Instead of talking only about polio vaccine, community workers in these areas also began to speak to mothers about the benefits of breast feeding and getting their children immunised for other diseases as well. They would also speak of the importance of hand washing, basic hygiene and the need to stop defecation in the open.

This broadening of the scope of the polio campaign was welcome. But many of the initiatives mentioned in the plan such as improving health and sanitation services remained on paper. While community workers were asked to talk to people about the importance of clean water and sanitation, and urge them to wash their hands, little was done to provide people with the means to achieve these goals. To be fair, improving sanitation and hygiene, providing clear drinking water and toilets were issues that the central and state governments in India had neglected for decades. It was unrealistic to expect the polio campaign to fix these issues. 'It would have made eradication easier if it brought broader benefits than polio,' admitted Hamid Jafari, the WHO's head of the polio programme in India during this period. 'But then it is a tall order…in a country with a population of one billion where 60 per cent have open defecation, how do you say let's improve sanitation before we work on eradication?'[11]

* * *

Stamping out the poliovirus from India showed that Albert Sabin's OPV could work its magic in the most difficult possible disease landscape. For the WHO and its partners in the campaign, it was seen as a vindication of its core belief that polio was an eradicable disease, and that this could be achieved without addressing more fundamental issues of sanitation and hygiene. It also seemed to demonstrate that even without a strong health system to deliver childhood vaccination, it was possible to eradicate polio by sending health workers out to knock on doors and deliver the vaccine. 'Questions about the vaccine were taken off the table, questions about sanitation and hygiene were taken off the table. It proved there was no technical or biological rationale for not achieving eradication. If it could be done in the setting of India, it could be done anywhere. It showed there was nothing wrong with the strategy,' said Hamid Jafari in an interview looking back at the experience.[12]

The end of polio in India was widely hailed as a landmark in the history of public health in India, alongside the eradication of smallpox. But like any victory, it came at a significant cost. The decade-long effort diverted attention away from other more essential health needs in India's poorest states. One study found that in Bihar, frontline government health workers were devoting more than seventy days a year to the polio campaign.[13] Researchers have attempted to quantify the impact that intensive polio campaigns have had on routine immunisation rates primary health care, but have not reached a definitive conclusion. In poor states accurate data is hard to come by, and it is hard to measure the full impact that intensive polio campaigns have on the health system, including the effects of fatigue on the part of health workers on the quality of the service they deliver.

The polio eradication campaign in India as elsewhere, also exposed the divide between a global health agenda set by such players as the WHO, other UN bodies and the Bill and Melinda Gates Foundation, and the interests of developing countries. India would not have chosen to spend the money it spent on stamping out the poliovirus unless it had been compelled to by international agencies. Polio was not a big enough problem on the Indian health agenda to justify the time and resources that went into it for nearly a decade and a half. And this was money and time that could have gone into other more urgent health issues.

The victory over polio in India has been rightly celebrated, but there are uncomfortable realities that have been swept under the carpet. Chief among them is the consistent brushing aside of the number of cases of children who were paralysed by the polio vaccine. Occasional cases of paralysis were a known side-effect of the Sabin vaccine. The WHO in its technical literature on the vaccine has estimated the risk of an infant developing paralysis from the vaccine as varying between one case per 1.4 million children in a birth cohort and one case per 2.8

million children. Another method of calculating the rate of vaccine-associated paralysis provides a figure of one case per 5.9 million doses administered. Sometimes, it was not the recipients of the vaccine, but their close contacts (usually a parent or sibling) who developed paralysis. Contact VAPP, as this is described, is estimated to occur at the rate of one case for every 6.7 million doses administered.

The risk appears tiny and the WHO consistently describes paralysis from the vaccine as very rare. But when a vaccine is administered on a scale that it was in India, the numbers are not insignificant. The WHO and the Indian government refuse to release any figures for vaccine associated paralysis, even though the WHO does keep a close tab. The only published figures are to be found in a study by a joint US CDC-WHO team led by Katherine Kohler of the US CDC. The study estimated that in India in 1999, there were 181 cases of paralysis caused by OPV with the age of the victims ranging from thirty seven days to thirty years Of these sixty cases were children who had received the vaccine themselves (recipient VAPP), while 120 cases were of children who had been infected after being in contact with someone who had received the vaccine (contact VAPP).[14] Kohler and her co-authors later updated these figures and estimated there were 129 cases in India in 2000 and 109 in 2001. They suggested that the figure of 181 in 1999 was unusually high because of a large number of children receiving a dose of OPV for the first time.[15]

The Enterovirus Research Institute in Mumbai, one of the country's premier research institutions and part of the WHO's network of polio laboratories, estimated in 2003–2004 between 91 and 208 cases of VAPP in under-fives in India.[16] This was a rare occasion on which a government laboratory provided figures for vaccine-associated paralysis in India, and it was never repeated again. Subsequent annual reports from the Enterovirus Research Centre, did not contain any figures for VAPP.

Since those early figures, the number of doses of polio vaccine administered every year in India have shot up dramatically. Each national immunisation day involves 172 million children receiving oral vaccine, and there are two of these each year. In addition, campaigns were held in Uttar Pradesh and Bihar and neighbouring states once every two months, vaccinating between 50–70 million children each time. This would push up the rate in the early studies.

A rule of thumb would be four to five cases per million births. With a birth cohort of 25 million births in India, that would result in a 100 to 125 children a year paralysed by the oral vaccine. This number would have reduced after April 2016 when the Type 2 component of the oral polio vaccine, which was known to cause a bulk of contact VAPP cases was withdrawn.[17]

Unlike in developed countries, where it was essential for parents to be warned of potential vaccination risks, and give informed consent before their children were vaccinated, in India there was no such requirement. Vaccinators would merely knock on doors, assure parents the vaccine was safe and pour drops into children's mouths. No one in the WHO, UNICEF, Rotary or the Bill and Melinda Gates Foundation broke the silence on this. Even the Indian Academy of Pediatrics, which was otherwise often critical of the polio programme, warned its members not to talk publicly about VAPP, lest the public lost confidence in the polio vaccine. 'The discussion on VAPP should be restricted to only academic circles' stated one position paper from the Academy.[18]

The elimination of the poliovirus has been one of global public health's famous victories. But, as is common whether in public health or in war, once the victory is won, the cost is quickly forgotten.

12

PAKISTAN

WHERE THE POLIOVIRUS HID IN BIN LADEN'S SHADOW

I landed at Benazir Bhutto International airport in Islamabad on a grey night in November 2014 and found myself in a country in crisis. The Pakistan government was under siege and paralysed. Over the past three months a charismatic cricketer turned politician, Imran Khan, and a cleric, Tahirul Qadri, had brought hundreds of thousands of protestors to Islamabad to force Prime Minister Nawaz Sharif to step down and hold fresh elections. A square known as D Chowk, overlooking the Prime Minister's official residence, had become the main protest site, the scene of fiery speeches and crowds chanting 'Go Nawaz Go'. The embattled Nawaz Sharif had refused to budge, and the protestors were refusing to lift their blockade of key government buildings, so there was talk of the army stepping in to declare martial law.

Newspapers and television stations reported the protests, as well as the other woes the nation faced, unsparingly. Along with the siege of the government, a six-month long military offensive against the Pakistan Taliban and its allies in the border areas of North Waziristan and Khyber had thrown over half a million people out of their homes. This river of displaced humanity was wending its way across the country, settling in camps, informal settlements and with friends and relatives. Others had crossed the border into Afghanistan. As a fallout of the action in the frontier regions, gun battles between the police and the Taliban had spread to Karachi, the country's commercial hub and its most cosmopolitan city. On a fairly typical day in November, three battles were reported between the police and militants in the poorer suburbs of Karachi. And there were the random acts of violence that characterise a society under stress. The day after I landed, the news was dominated by the horrific killing of a Christian couple from a village near Lahore who had been beaten and burned alive in a brick kiln after being accused of desecrating the Koran.

Two months earlier, in September, nature had compounded Pakistan's man-made woes when four major rivers, the Ravi, the Chenab, the Jhelum and the Sutlej, swollen by torrential rains, burst their banks and destroyed homes, crops, fields and animals, affecting nearly 2 million people. The cash-strapped Pakistan government had asked donors for US$2.5 million to repair flood damage and help rehabilitate those who had lost their homes in the military operations in North Waziristan.

In the midst of these multiple challenges, the Pakistan government faced another crisis; not one that threatened its grip on domestic power, but one that was vastly damaging to its international reputation. Pakistan at the end of 2014 was one of the last few places on earth where polio existed. After a campaign that had been proceeding in fits and starts since 1988, the goal of eradicating polio globally appeared to be in sight. Pakistan was polio's last frontier. While in Nigeria and Afghanistan, the two other countries where polio was endemic, the numbers of cases had dwindled to the single figures, in Pakistan cases were rising, seemingly uncontrollably. Over 250 cases were recorded that year, the highest in the country in at least a decade.

The rising polio cases were a symptom of Pakistan's deeper malaise. The poor governance and endemic corruption fuelling protests against Sharif were also why an act as simple as immunising children under the age of five twice a year with two drops of OPV had proved impossible to achieve. The violence, apathy and mutual distrust between government and people that ran like threads through the fabric of Pakistani society, was clear to see in the polio programme's struggles.

The relationship between the Pakistan government and the polio programme plunged to a new low in May 2014 after the Independent Monitoring Board (IMB) of the polio programme had delivered a scathing report on Pakistan's performance. In language free of diplomatic obfuscation, and with a directness rarely seen in the world of global health diplomacy, the report said 'Pakistan's polio programme is a disaster. It continues to flounder helplessly as its virus flourishes.'[1] The IMB report described Pakistan as the major stumbling block to global polio eradication, and described the country as 'a real and present danger to people in neighbouring countries and farther afield.' The IMB's members were independent of the WHO and the polio programme, but the report was seen as based on briefings that WHO and the other polio partners had provided to the IMB.

The report was a humiliation for the government, and marked the second time that polio had been a cause for international embarrassment. A year earlier the WHO had used the International Health Regulations to require Pakistanis travelling abroad to be vaccinated against polio so they did not spread the disease abroad. Pakistan's elite was outraged at the thought that they were being considered carriers of disease, while the poor took this as another in the endless series of humiliations they were required to endure. And they all blamed the government for heaping this indignity on them.

Government officials fumed in private at what they saw as a refusal by the IMB and the WHO to recognise the challenges that Pakistan faced in eradicating polio. I went to see Mazhar Nisar Sheikh, a former television journalist who had trained in public health and was now a senior official in the Federal Ministry of Health. When I walked into his cramped office in the early afternoon, he was trying to eat a hurried lunch of rice and dhal out of a plastic box and affably offered me some. A stream of people came in and out of the room, some with requests, some merely to say hello, and some who had dropped in because they had seemingly little else to do. His phone rang incessantly. At one stage, he rushed out of the room in response to one of the calls. 'That was my Minister,' he explained apologetically when he returned.

When he got to talking about polio, Mazhar let it be known the government was affronted by the report and its description of Pakistani ineptitude. Pakistan's situation was unique, he said. Polio vaccinators, the lowest paid and most vulnerable link in the polio programme, were being assassinated by the Pakistan Taliban and its allies as they went house-to-house immunising children. In the last three years, sixty-four polio workers had been killed this way, several of them women. Nowhere else in the world had polio vaccinators been targeted and assassinated as they had been in Pakistan. 'The international community should understand the geopolitical environment in which we operate,' he said. 'We have told them that we will do our best, but we will not be dictated to'.

A day later, I met with Elias Durry, the Ethiopian-born head of the WHO's polio campaign in Pakistan. Durry is an intense, driven, bull of a man, who had negotiated his way through the fraught and violent tribal politics of Somalia to eradicate polio in that country before being put in charge of Pakistan. He is a chain smoker, so we sat at an outdoor terrace at his hotel on a bright, but chilly morning. As he puffed on cigarettes and sipped coffee, Durry did little to hide his frustration with the Pakistani government. 'We understand the problems caused by the killings, the problems caused by the military operations…but when you have a strong government and the fourth largest army in the world, how come you cannot manage these things?'

Durry found Somalia, with its lawlessness and lack of government easier to deal with than Pakistan. 'In Somalia, there is no system, here there is a system that is against you,' he says. He recounts numerous instances where polio campaigns have had to be cancelled because the police escorts failed to turn up on time. 'In other countries during campaigns we used to go from the health outpost to health outpost to see if things were OK. Here we go from police station to police station to see if they have sent enough police to the field. This should not be our job.'

Durry was still optimistic that polio could be brought under control in Pakistan. All it required was four or five well implemented immunisation rounds in the first half of the year (the polio low season) for the disease to be stopped in its tracks. And it was not even as though polio was a problem all over in the country. It was only a handful of areas: the tribal areas bordering Afghanistan, the province of Khyber Pakhtunkhwa, and Karachi where the poliovirus persisted. 'If we can hit all of these regions with good campaigns simultaneously, we can do it.'

Listening to Durry, I was once again reminded of the huge gap between the optimistic assumptions with which the polio eradication campaign had been launched in 1988 and the reality in places like

Pakistan, plagued by civil strife, bureaucratic inertia and public apathy. If that was not enough, Pakistan was also where the polio programme found itself caught in the crossfire of the war between the United States and the Islamic fundamentalist armies inspired by Osama bin Laden.

* * *

On a Tuesday morning in July 2012 at around mid-day, a white Datsun pickup truck was negotiating its way through the crowded streets of Sohrab Goth in Karachi. Suddenly two gunmen on a motorcycle rode up, shot the truck's tyres to force it to a halt, and then turned their attention to the occupants inside. Constant Dedo, a Ghanaian doctor with the WHO's polio programme, received a bullet in his abdomen, while his local driver was shot in the shoulder. Both were taken to one of Karachi's best-equipped hospitals, the Aga Khan Hospital, where they recovered. The shooting happened on the second day of a three-day polio immunisation campaign, and while no one claimed responsibility for the killings, the attacks were widely perceived to be if not directly carried out by, at the very least inspired by, the Pakistan Taliban.

The shots that rang out on that dusty road in Karachi were not the first warning that the Taliban had delivered to the polio eradication campaign. Nor were they to be the last.

On 18 December that year, two women vaccinators, 18-year-old Madiha Shah, and her aunt Fehmida Shah, dressed in the black burkhas they habitually wore outside their houses and collected their distinctive blue vaccine boxes. They slung them across their shoulders and set off through the narrow lanes of Gulshan-e-Buner a predominantly Pashtun locality in eastern Karachi. There had been threats against polio workers before, but the two women were close to home. There were also other women in the family on the vaccination team: Madiha's mother Ruksana and her aunt Gulnaz, who was a supervisor of the team. A day earlier, a male vaccinator had been shot dead on the first day of the campaign in Gadap, a few kilometres away. But there was no police protection for the vaccinators, who went ahead with their day's work regardless. The women had apparently faced abuse earlier while doing their rounds. 'Men used to hurl abuse at us saying we were engaged in a drive aimed at spreading infertility', their relatives told the *Dawn* newspaper.[2]

They needed the money. Madiha's father, had had an operation recently and could not work. Madiha and Ruksana were the breadwinners of the family, and the Rs. 250 a day (roughly US$2.50) they were paid was a pittance even by Pakistani standards, but it helped to keep the family afloat. Fehmida had seven children, and her husband Syed, was a daily wage worker.

Around noon, as Madiha and Fehmida were knocking on a door to see if there were any children that could be vaccinated, a motorcycle with two men on it drove up to them, and one man took out a gun and shot both women. Madiha fell immediately, but Fehmida managed to scramble to a nearby doorway, where one of the assassins followed her and shot her repeatedly.[3] Madiha's mother Ruksana was in another house administering drops, and when she came out, she saw a man holding a gun. She ran and escaped, not knowing her daughter had been shot. More was to come. In what were clearly planned and coordinated attacks, Naseema Akhtar, a vaccinator doing her rounds in nearby Orangi town was shot dead in a similar manner about fifteen minutes later while a male colleague was critically injured. Around the same time, another woman vaccinator, Kaneez Jan was shot dead in nearby Itehaad town. A male vaccinator she was with was injured but survived.[4] On the same day in Peshawar in northwest Pakistan, a 17-year-old girl, Farzana Bibi was shot dead while administering vaccine, and a day later a woman supervisor of the vaccination campaign and her driver were killed in a district outside Peshawar. In the space of three days, nine vaccinators, all but one of them women, were shot dead in perhaps the most brutal attack than any health campaign has ever had to face.[5]

As the families of the dead collapsed in grief, the WHO reeled with the horror of what had happened. This was not the first time a global health campaign had been caught in the midst of civil strife. In places like Somalia, the polio vaccinators had to negotiate with warring clan leaders to be allowed to vaccinate children. In Peru, the WHO had to negotiate days of tranquillity between the government and the Shining Path guerrilla movement for vaccinators to immunise children. But in all of these cases, the vaccinators were not part of the conflict: they were seen as disinterested humanitarian workers, and the warring parties respected this and gave them space to work. However in Pakistan it was different. The polio eradication campaign itself was the target in a wider war, a bystander that had stumbled into a conflict, found itself taken hostage, and then turned into a target.

PAKISTAN

The killing of vaccinators raised an ethical issue that no health campaigns had yet confronted: what price in human lives was the polio campaign willing to tolerate in order to finish the job? As Heidi Larson of the London School of Hygiene and Tropical Medicine commented, 'More people are dying as vaccinators than have from polio. There's something wrong with that equation.'[6] After the attacks in 2012, the polio campaign suspended vaccination campaigns in areas where their teams were at risk. But after persuading the local police and the army to provide better security, the campaigns gradually resumed, even though the attacks against vaccinators continued.

Between 2012 and 2017, over 100 vaccinators as well as policemen on security duty during vaccinations have been shot dead. During most of 2013 and for most of 2014 as well, vaccination campaigns were suspended in parts of Karachi, the tribal areas of North and South Waziristan, and in areas around Peshawar, the capital of the province of Khyber Pakhtunkhwa. The number of cases of polio in the country shot up from 58 in 2012 to 306 in 2014, a year in which Pakistan accounted for 85 per cent of the global cases of polio. Violence and the bans by the Taliban were not the only reason for the rise in cases. Polio campaigns in parts of Pakistan had been poorly run by provincial governments and local governments, and corruption and a general lack of urgency felt by local and provincial health authorities all contributed to the persistence of polio in Pakistan. But the most obvious and easily discernible reason for the persistence of polio in Pakistan during this period, was the shadow cast by the Taliban. That was not least because of the way the polio campaign was ensnared in the hunt for Osama bin Laden

* * *

The tribulations of the polio eradication campaign in Pakistan are often portrayed as a reflection of Islamic fundamentalism, and as an example of the Taliban's ruthlessness in holding the health of children hostage in their pursuit of power. That is partly true. But to understand the spider's web that the polio eradication campaign became trapped in, it is also important to delve below the surface of events. The Taliban in Pakistan, the religious leaders who fuelled and supported them, the often dysfunctional Pakistan government, and the all-powerful Pakistan military, were all players in a dangerous game. This game was being played against the backdrop of the longest running geo-political conflict that the world has seen since the end of the Cold War. It was in Pakistan, more than anywhere else in the world that the managers of the polio eradication campaign had to develop skills that they had never been taught in medical school. They had to learn to wend their way between warring parties and factions within Pakistani society and build alliances with opposition political parties while still keeping the government on board. Beyond this they had to woo the Pakistan military without whose support nothing of importance can happen in Pakistan and reach out to Islamic preachers. At the same time they had to ensure that repeated polio vaccination campaigns were carried out by an overstretched health service that for the most part had little interest in focusing all its attention on polio.

Pakistan is where the polio campaign, conceived and planned in the meeting rooms of the WHO's headquarters in the serene surroundings of Geneva, Switzerland, had to confront a stark reality. It had to carry out its public health mission in a country that was crumbling from the pressure of being on the frontline of the war between Islamic fundamentalism and the Western world.

It was not clear what prompted the Taliban in Pakistan to turn their attention to polio immunisation. In 2006, a preacher from the Swat Valley in Pakistan's frontier area, Maulana Fazlullah, who would later head the Pakistan Taliban, took aim at the polio eradication campaign, describing the vaccination drives as a 'conspiracy of the Jews and Christians to stunt the growth of Muslims'. The Maulana did not indicate what led him to this conclusion, but he told the BBC that if international organisations were keen on helping Muslims, they should do something about hepatitis instead, which was a bigger health threat.[7]

In another interview to a local news website in Swat, Fazlullah added an objection based on his interpretation of Sharia law, and also demanded wider health care from the government. 'To cure a disease before its onset is not in accordance with Sharia's laws. The relevant experts have also questioned the credibility of the polio vaccine... Why the government looks to be so much interested in this affair, there are so many other fatal diseases which are too much costly to be treated. The government should provide people free medical facilities to relieve them from financial burden.'[8]

The narrative linking polio vaccine to a Western conspiracy to harm Muslims was first heard in Nigeria in 2003. Five northern Nigerian states with predominantly Muslim populations decided to boycott the polio vaccine. This was after several influential leaders declared the polio vaccine to be part of the West's revenge for the 9/11 attacks, and were designed to spread HIV and make Muslim children infertile. These claims first appear to have been made by local preachers and religious leaders. But they gained traction after the head of the Sharia Council of Nigeria, a practising doctor by name Dr Datti Ahmad, made a declaration based on documents he had seen. 'We believe that modern day Hitlers have deliberately adulterated the oral polio vaccines with anti-fertility drugs and contaminated it with certain viruses which are known to cause HIV and AIDS,' he said.[9] The campaign against the vaccine occurred shortly after the US invasion of Iraq, and with war in Afghanistan continuing, there was a perception among Muslims of a Western, Christian war against Islam. A spokesman for Kano state in Nigeria, Sule Ya'u expressed this when he said, 'Since September 11, the Muslim world is beginning to be suspicious of any move from the Western world. Our people have really become concerned about polio vaccine.'[10]

The WHO enlisted the aid of prominent Islamic scholars and launched an enormous publicity campaign to convince the Muslim population of Northern Nigeria that the vaccines did not call any of the ills ascribed to it. The same narrative around the vaccine popped up again in Pakistan, propagated across the radio waves by a firebrand preacher on a bootleg radio station. In Pakistan, these rumours about the vaccine fell on an audience that was perhaps even more receptive than in Nigeria. While the wars in Iraq and Afghanistan were distant events in Nigeria, for those living in the border areas between Pakistan and Afghanistan, the war was a daily reality. For the population of the frontier areas of Pakistan, the coming and going of armed Taliban fighters across the border with Pakistan, and the US drone attacks on suspected Taliban targets had become part of their lives. The United States and the West was the enemy, and it was easy to see why a vaccination programme that was funded by global organisations was seen with suspicion, particularly when no other form of health care reached these areas.

The Taliban took the campaign against the vaccine a step further by linking them to the drone attacks the US was carrying out in Pakistan on suspected Taliban targets. One of the largest such attacks happened in October 2006, when a madrassa in Chenagai village in the frontier region of Bajaur in Pakistan was hit by missiles. It is not clear who the target was, but eighty-two people—many of them local students—were killed, much to the outrage of the public. The United States was widely thought to be behind the strike, since it had carried out similar strikes earlier. That included one earlier that year in the village of Damadola, also in Bajaur, on a building where the then al Qaeda Number 2, Ayman Al Zawahiri, was thought to be. Neither Al-Zawahiri nor any other senior al Qaeda leaders were in the building, but a number of civilians were believed killed. All of this increased public anger, and allowed the Taliban to introduce a new narrative. The vaccinators were actually spies for the Americans, and were being used to gather intelligence on Taliban and al Qaeda movements and indicate targets for drone attacks. No one knows to what extent people in Pakistan bought this argument when it was first made in 2006. But it rapidly became credible in the public mind after the events of 1 May 2011. This was the night Osama bin Laden was killed by Navy SEAL commandos in the town of Abbottabad, a three-and-a-half-hour drive from the seat of the Pakistani government in Islamabad.

The tracking of Bin Laden is a fascinating story. It led to a lot of soul searching in Pakistan. How was it possible for one of the world's most wanted men to live in the country from around 2002, spending the last six years of his life in Abbottabad, a town where the Pakistan military had a significant presence? (Bin Laden's hideout was just 1 kilometre as the crow flies from the Pakistan Military Academy, the training ground for the country's future military officers).

But for our purposes, what is relevant is the way in which the US hunt for Bin Laden intersected with the global hunt for the poliovirus. The CIA used many methods to try and establish Bin Laden's presence in Abbottabad. One was the recruitment of a Pakistani doctor, Dr Shakeel Afridi, to conduct a vaccination campaign among children in the area around the house that Bin Laden was believed to be hiding. This was in the hope that the needles used for vaccination would contain DNA samples that could be used to establish whether Bin Laden's family lived in the house.

The DNA evidence that the CIA was hoping to get out of the campaign did not materialise, since the women and children of the Bin Laden family did not get themselves vaccinated. Afridi maintains he had no idea that the vaccination campaign was sponsored by the CIA, or what its objective was. As far as he was concerned, he was asked by an international NGO to help carry out a hepatitis B vaccination campaign, and that was all he did. If he had been a CIA operative, or felt he had done something wrong, he would have fled the country immediately, rather than wait around to be captured nearly a month after the event.

There is no doubt that Afridi was used by the CIA (the only doubt can be over how much he himself was aware that he was being used.) The US government itself acknowledged Afridi's role, and called for his release. Speaking after Afridi was sentenced to thirty-three years in prison, Leon Panetta, the CIA Director at the time of the Abbottabad raid told an interviewer that, 'It is so difficult to understand and it's so disturbing that they would sentence this doctor to thirty-three years for helping in the search for the most notorious terrorist of our times...This doctor was not working against Pakistan, he was working against al Qaeda.'[11] The then US Secretary of State, Hillary Clinton, also described the sentence as 'unjust and unwarranted', while US Senators voted to cut US$33 billion of US aid to Pakistan—US$1 billion for every year of Afridi's sentence.

The CIA's use of a vaccination programme to help in the hunt for Bin Laden was to have an enormous impact on polio eradication programme. The mullahs and Taliban leaders who had been railing against polio vaccinators and describing them as US spies, now seemed to have been justified in their suspicions. It did not help that once news of Afridi's arrest and his role in the raid on Bin Laden broke, many news reports described Afridi as having conducted a polio vaccination programme sponsored by the CIA. Parents who had wavered earlier about whether to vaccinate their children seem to have had their doubts confirmed.

Taliban leaders began to issue fresh bans on polio vaccination, drawing explicit links to the CIA's use of Shakil Afridi. In June 2012, a month before the WHO's Dr Constant Dedo was shot in Karachi, Hafiz Gul, a Taliban commander in North Waziristan published a decree on behalf of a Higher Council of Mujahideen calling for a complete ban on polio vaccination. 'There is a high possibility that the campaign be used for spying against the Mujahideen. An apt example for this is Dr Shakil Afridi. Therefore, there shall be a total ban on the anti-polio drive.'[12]

Gul's declaration also called for a ban on drone attacks as a condition for allowing polio vaccination to continue. 'Polio infects one child in a million, but hundreds of Waziri women, children and elders have been killed in these strikes.' The drone attacks were also causing psychological problems in the population. 'Each day the list of psychological patients increases in Waziristan, which is worse than polio.'

Gul's edict came at a time when the CIA had stepped up the intensity of its drone attacks in Pakistan. Data compiled by the UK-based Bureau of Investigative Journalists showed that drone strikes had reached new levels of intensity in the early summer of 2012.[13] In the last week of May, there had been four attacks in six days, including on a bakery in the town of Miranshah in North Waziristan that had apparently been used by al Qaeda and Taliban figures. The attacks seemed to be targeting senior al Qaeda leaders (Abu Yahya al Libi, described as the effective Number 2 in al Qaeda, was among those killed in early June in North Waziristan). The Pakistan Taliban could well have decided to hit back by targeting what seemed to them to be an aid programme backed by the US and run largely by Westerners. (This was even though the victims of the Taliban assassinations were always local men and women vaccinators.)

While the local Taliban leaders were often at odds with the traditional tribal leadership, the ban announced by Hafiz Gul was echoed by a jirga of tribal elders. They decided to refuse polio immunisation until the government provided their villages with electricity. One of the leaders, Malik Mashal Khan was quoted in a newspaper report as saying, 'If our children die from the scorching heat and mosquito bites, so what if they die of polio. We will continue the boycott until the government fulfils our demand. We are betrayed with false promises of the government and the officials are doing nothing practical.'[14]

Later in the same month, another Taliban group in neighbouring South Waziristan, the Mullah Nazir group, called for a similar ban on polio vaccination and linked a resumption of immunisation to an ending of drone attacks. A pamphlet distributed in the region compared polio vaccine to 'sugar coated poison' and asked 'If they (the United States and its allies) were so sincere with the Muslims, then why did they bomb us so mercilessly?'[15]

More than the drone attacks, the use of Shakil Afridi by the CIA was a wound from which the polio programme would take a long time to recover. Dr Zulfikar Ahmad Bhutta, a public health and vaccine special-ist at Aga Khan University in Karachi did not mince words about the impact of the Afridi affair 'There could not have been a more stupid venture, and there was bound to be a backlash, especially for polio.'[16] Senior figures in the polio programme who visited the frontier areas to talk to the Taliban, found Afridi at the top of every conversation. 'All the parents I talked to mentioned the vaccinations that Afridi had con-ducted for the CIA, and were suspicious', recalls Aziz Memon, the head of the Rotary's polio efforts in Pakistan.[17]

The WHO and the polio campaign as a whole was powerless to distance itself, or in any way condemn the use of a health programme to conduct espionage. This was even though the WHO had been receiv-ing advice from religious as well as community leaders to publicly state its opposition to the use of health campaigns for other purposes. But the WHO was unable to do this. The United States was the WHO's major funder (there has never been an instance where the WHO has issued any kind of rebuke to the United States on any issue). The US CDC, which was part of the US government, was one of the partners in the US polio eradication campaign. Two other partners, Rotary International and the Gates Foundation, were US-based organisations that were reluctant to publicly condemn the US government, particu-larly when CIA programme was aimed at capturing Osama bin Laden.

Nim'a Saeed Abid, an Iraqi born physician who was head of the WHO's polio programme at the time of the attacks felt that the WHO had a moral responsibility to say that public health programmes should not be used for anything other than public health. But he also said there was no appetite in the WHO's leadership in Geneva to take a stand on this. In 2014 though, Nim'a Abid, in his capacity as acting head of the WHO office in Islamabad made the WHO's first and only public rebuke for the CIA's use of a vaccination campaign in the hunt for Bin Laden. 'The improper use of vaccination campaigns by certain agencies has adversely affected public health activities in the region, leading to declining participation of the locals,' he said at a news conference. Abid got permission for what he was going to say from the WHO's regional director in Cairo, Ala Alawan (perhaps knowing that WHO headquar-ters in Geneva would not be supportive).[18]

Ultimately, it was a group of influential deans from schools of public health in the United States who spoke out against the use of a vaccination campaign by the CIA, and won an undertaking from the CIA not to use such methods again. The deans of twelve schools of public health in the United States wrote a strongly worded letter to President Obama in January 2013. In it they said that 'contaminating humanitarian and public health programs with covert activities threatens the present participants and future potential of what we undertake internationally to improve health and provide humanitarian assistance.' They urged Obama to 'assure the public that this type of practice will not be repeated.'[19] Obama responded to the Deans through a letter from Homeland Security Lisa Monaco stating that in August 2013, the CIA Director, John Brennan, had issued an order forbidding the agency from using vaccination programmes to gather intelligence.[20]

The problems that the polio programme faced in Pakistan were of course not solely due to the CIA's vaccination programme. The Taliban in Pakistan had issued bans on polio vaccination and killed vaccinators in the border regions well before the raid on Bin Laden. If anything, the US drone attacks on Taliban leaders in Pakistan were a more important cause for the ban on vaccinators. But even if the US had stopped drone attacks, there was no guarantee that the Taliban would change its mind on polio vaccination. That was because the ban on vaccinations was also part of a wider anger within the Taliban about the role that women were playing in the vaccination campaign.

When the Taliban came to power in Afghanistan one of their first acts was to remove women from all public life and public activity. They confined them to their homes, and allowed them to emerge in public only if they were suitably escorted and covered and shielded from male gaze. When the Taliban in Pakistan took control of Pakistan's frontier regions, they followed their Afghan colleagues in restricting the public life of women. Afiya Sherbano Zia writes that during the Taliban's three-year rule over Swat in the frontier region, they destroyed 165 girls' schools, in addition to banning music and cinema. The most visible area in which women performed public functions was in health care. Pakistan had a cadre of female community health workers known as Lady Health Workers, who had been created to deliver health services to the community, including polio vaccination and family planning. The Lady Health Workers became a particular target of the Taliban, and fatwas were issued banning them from work.[21]

A report in the *British Medical Journal*, based on accounts from people living in Swat, exposed the harassment to which women health workers were exposed.[22] One fatwa declared that the presence of women in public spaces was a form of public indecency. It stated that it was a Muslim man's duty to kidnap women health workers when they made home visits and marry them forcibly, even if they were already married. The Taliban would visit the homes of women health workers and threaten their families with beheading if the women continued to work. One health supervisor in the region recounted 'The Taliban would come. They would call their (LHW's) brothers or fathers to the door. They used very bad language about the girls...the brothers cannot tolerate such language against their sisters. So they argued back—that is their job—the Taliban just killed them.'[23]

The Taliban's vicious anger against women health workers seemed to stem from three causes: they were women; they were also involved in distributing contraceptives and giving family planning advice to women (contraception was considered un-Islamic by the Taliban); and they were also the front line of the polio campaign, which the Taliban was using as a tool to gain leverage with the US to stop drone attacks.

Women were essential to the polio immunisation campaign. Men could not gain access to homes where, as was very often the case during the day, the men had gone out and there were only women and children. It took years of effort to recruit women into the vaccination campaign after persuading fathers, husbands and brothers to allow their female family members to work. By targeting women, the Taliban effectively targeted both the most vulnerable, as well as the most essential link in the chain that delivered polio vaccines to children.

Many women, with their lives under threat, and with children and family to care for, decided the risks were too great until the threat from the Taliban ended. The report on conditions in Swat published in the *BMJ*, noted that around 15 per cent of women health workers resigned, while others gradually stopped working. Others publicly burned the health brochures and pamphlets that they used to distribute, in order to announce they were no longer part of the Lady Health Workers programme. Some moved out of Swat.

The polio campaign treated the Taliban's propaganda as well as physical attacks on the polio programme as the result of misconceptions among Islamic fundamentalists about the nature of the poliovirus. And in order to change these misconceptions, it enlisted the services of other Islamic scholars and imams. It asked them to certify that the polio vaccine contained no harmful or 'haram' substances, that it was not un-Islamic to vaccinate children, and that polio vaccine was not intended to render Muslim children sterile. Imams were enlisted to mention the benefits of polio vaccine in their Friday sermons; religious figures were persuaded to publicly feed polio drops to their children. The Ulema Council, an umbrella group of scholars representing different Muslim sects voiced its support for polio eradication. Beyond this a plethora of groups with a variety of titles, funded by the polio programme through a variety of sources including donations from the UAE, were set up to advocate in favour of immunisation. These included an Islamic Advisory Task Force, a Religious Support Persons and Provincial Scholars Task Force, and an Urban Council Task Force, bodies which met at regular intervals to issue proclamations in favour of polio immunisation.

But the opposition to vaccination was not religious; it was political. Except for Nigeria and the Taliban in Pakistan, and certain pockets in Uttar Pradesh in India, nowhere else in the Islamic world was there any religious opposition to vaccination. Saudi Arabia, the guardian of the holiest sites in Islam, had in fact made it mandatory for pilgrims entering the country to be vaccinated against polio. Even the Taliban in Afghanistan did not block polio immunisation. (The problem in Afghanistan was more about providing access to vaccination teams in conflict areas, rather than any religious objection.) The majority of the Islamic world, with the exception of Pakistan and Nigeria, had been polio-free for decades, and conducted annual polio immunisation campaigns without encountering any religious hurdles.

In Pakistan, the poliovirus proved to be a bit player in a wider game involving the Pakistan government, the Pakistan army, the Taliban and the United States. Of all the pieces on the chessboard, the Pakistan military (which sees itself as the ultimate guarantor of the Pakistani state and has deposed civilian governments on several occasions in the country's history) was the key. It could free the frontier regions from the Taliban, and allow the vaccination teams to resume their work. The army in Pakistan had a complex relationship with the Taliban. The military had been involved in training and nurturing the Taliban, which it saw as a way of extending Pakistani influence in Afghanistan. But at the same time, the Taliban were an unreliable partner; their war against the United States, and their determination to bring in Sharia Law to the tribal areas and then the rest of Pakistan put them at odds with the military. Clashes between the military and the Taliban intensified, with the Taliban launching increasingly bold attacks outside its traditional tribal strongholds. These included an attack on Jinnah International Airport in Karachi in June 2014 in which over thirty people died. In the same month, the military decided to act, and began an operation named Zarb e Azb, the largest military campaign it had ever conducted to clear the tribal areas of the Taliban, beginning in North and South Waziristan. A Taliban suicide attack on an army school in Peshawar in December 2014 that killed 132 school children removed whatever hesitancy the army might have had in going after the Taliban.

As thousands of Waziris fled the fighting and crossed to other provinces, the polio campaign finally found a way to reach children it had been unable to for the last several years. As the children and their families streamed out, polio vaccination points were established at transit points including railway stations and bus terminals across the country to try and vaccinate children. Elias Durry, the head of the WHO polio programme in Pakistan, was pleased with the progress when I spoke to him six months after the Pakistan army had launched its operation. 'At least 80 per cent of the children of North Waziristan are now reachable…this is a complete change from eighteen months back.'

Once it began action against the Taliban, the army also became more amenable to the idea of providing security to polio vaccinators, something it had been reluctant to do earlier. Aziz Memon, who led Rotary's polio initiative in Pakistan, observed that it had been essential to get army backing for the polio programme if it was to succeed in the frontier areas. 'How can we immunise children who are totally under the control of the militants? It is not possible unless the army comes in and clears the areas first.'

Memon, who is a wealthy, well-connected Karachi businessman, had lobbied to get greater army security for vaccinators. This included at one stage dropping in on former President Parvez Musharraf at his home in Karachi and urging him to use his influence in the Army to get

POLIO

them involved in helping the polio campaign. Speaking in early 2015, six months after the military operations against the Taliban had begun, Memon said 'security is still a concern, but the army is now openly supporting us, unlike before.'[24]

In mid-2017, three years after operation Zarb e Azb was launched, the Taliban had been dislodged from large parts of Pakistan's border areas. It had not disappeared but had withdrawn to safe areas across the Afghan border, from where they return to ambush army patrols and lay landmines. But they were no longer in a position ban vaccination, and there were only a few isolated pockets in the tribal areas that were still off limits to the polio campaign. However the virus still circulates in the frontier areas, from where it is carried to Afghanistan and other parts of Pakistan. Like the Taliban, it has retreated, but has not gone away, and as the Taliban resurfaces to attack the Army, the poliovirus resurfaces periodically to cripple children. The deeper reasons for the poliovirus' resilience, lies in the dysfunction of the Pakistani state, as well as the great divide between what the polio programme was doing, and what the people of Pakistan actually needed in terms of health care.

* * *

'We used to say polio eradication is triple twos: two drops, two stool samples, in two weeks', mused Durry, who was managing the Pakistan polio programme in that difficult period after the 2012 killings of vaccinators by the Taliban in Karachi and Peshawar. 'Two drops twice a year to eliminate, the virus, and two stool samples taken with a two-week gap to confirm whether a case of paralysis is caused by polio.'

Even without vaccinators getting killed, these simple tasks presuppose the existence of a functioning health system with the ability and the desire to carry out these tasks. Pakistan is country with a well-trained class of professionals, a system of government inherited from its days as a British colony that provided a robust framework for health care delivery. So on paper, Pakistan was more than capable of eliminating polio. But there was never a very convincing reason for either the federal or the provincial governments (in Pakistan provincial governments had ultimate responsibility for health) to devote the kind of attention and resources required to stamp out polio in the face of a wealth of other competing demands. This was especially so when a government was fighting for political survival (as the Nawaz Sharif government was from 2014 onward), and polio eradication was not essential to helping it to survive. Fighting an armed insurgency as well as prolonged opposition protests that were paralysing the government, polio was low on the list of essential things to do. The previous Pakistan People's Party government, led by Asif Zardari, the husband of the assassinated Benazir Bhutto, had been receptive to the idea of polio eradication. Zardari's sister, Azra Pechuho, a doctor by training, headed a committee to oversee the government's polio campaign. But after an election brought a new government headed by Nawaz Sharif into power, the momentum was lost. It took sustained pressure from the WHO and the other partners in the eradication campaign to get the government to pay attention to polio.

The WHO has only one way to put pressure on governments. That is by invoking the International Health Regulations (IHR) which are legally binding on the WHO's member countries. In 2014, the WHO Director General, Margaret Chan, convened an emergency committee under the IHR. She declared polio to be an international public health emergency based on the international spread of poliovirus from Pakistan, Syria and Cameroon, and required that everyone from these countries travelling abroad be given a dose of polio vaccine. The real target of these measures was Pakistan. The outbreaks in Syria and Cameroon were short-term and could be stamped out soon. The impact of the requirement to ensure that all travellers leaving Pakistan were vaccinated was probably debatable on public health grounds. Travellers from Pakistan had carried poliovirus to the Middle East and Xinjiang in China. There was also a constant movement of the poliovirus across the soft border between Afghanistan and Pakistan. But it was not clear to what extent giving travellers polio drops (particularly at airport departure areas) would stop them spreading the virus. No studies had been conducted on the role of adults in transmitting poliovirus. Nor had there been studies on how effective a single dose of OPV would be in stopping an adult from transmitting poliovirus. Zulfikar Ahmed Bhutta, a professor at the Aga Khan University in Karachi, wrote in a commentary published in *Nature* that 'vaccinating travellers will be ineffective, and it could make polio harder to eliminate in the poor and conflict-ridden parts of Pakistan.'[25]

Bhutta pointed out that there were roughly 7 million Pakistanis working overseas, mostly as labourers in the Middle East. He said that getting them all immunised would be a distraction from the wider task of immunising children in the frontier areas, the main driver of polio transmission in Pakistan.

The WHO's demand that Pakistanis travelling abroad needed to get vaccinated against polio may not have made much sense from the public health perspective. But politically, it was an astute move that quickly forced government attention on the polio campaign. Perhaps even more importantly, it focused public attention on the failure to eradicate polio. The immediate impact of the WHO's recommendation were frantic queues at airports, where makeshift counters had been set up for departing travellers who needed to get last minute polio drops. Hospitals and clinics were besieged by travellers wanting polio drops and certificates to prove they had been immunised. A report in the *Dawn* newspaper by two journalists who visited the vaccination counter at Islamabad airport found unruly queues, short tempers, shortages of vaccines and panicky travellers.[26]

News reports from the provinces indicated confusion about where the extra vaccine supplies that would be required for travellers was to come from, and who was to pay for it, with provincial health departments baulking at the extra strain on their health budgets.

The Pakistan government was angry at the restrictions but it was also stung into action. The Prime Minister, Nawaz Sharif, summoned a meeting of provincial chief ministers as well as his own senior ministers, and declared that he would deliver a polio-free Pakistan in six months and would supervise the campaign personally. 'Polio epidemic will not be tolerated in this country....I refuse to put the generations of Pakistan at risk.'[27]

Regardless of such declarations from the Prime Minister, little was actually happening on the ground. There were multiple crises ranging from military action in the north-west frontier, to power shortages and floods that Pakistan was facing at the time. This meant there was neither the time nor the energy in the government to focus on polio. Polio eradication was not going to bail Nawaz Sharif from his various political predicaments, nor was it a sufficiently important issue in Pakistani domestic politics to be a vote winner for him at the next election. 'You have to understand why people voted for this government. People voted for them to control terrorism, electricity and so on,' remarked Babar bin Atta, a political and communication consultant in Islamabad.

Durry was determined to do whatever it took to get the polio programme in Pakistan going again. If the federal government was not interested, then he decided he would go directly to the provinces. 'At the end of the day, the work is done at the local level. So we started going to the district commissioners and union councils and help them with planning. We also work closely with the provinces, and we go talk to the Chief Ministers and senior government officials and advocate for change in the way the campaign is managed.' In the process, the WHO role began to change from a technical organisation providing advice to governments, to an implementing agency. 'People say this is a WHO run programme, but that is the only way to do this in the absence of strong government leadership,' Durry observed.[28]

Durry had been sent to Pakistan by the polio programme in Geneva in 2012 to get the polio programme moving in the country. In the process he ruffled feathers. A major weakness was the leakage of money through corruption and inefficiency, which left frontline polio workers unpaid for long periods of time. 'The polio programme has been going on for sixteen years and it had been going on for so long that it had become its own enemy, and it created its own mafia,' he said. The WHO found that in Karachi, one of the hot spots for polio in the country, half the names listed as vaccinators were children under the age of fifteen. These were clearly ghost vaccinators, and the money was being pocketed by people in the system. 'This was no longer a small programme, and people could become, I don't know, millionaires in a few years.' Corruption was an open secret, but nothing was being done about it.

'Everybody saw this, and no one was saying anything. The problem was also of our own making. We used to pay money to the district health department, and they would give it to supervisors, and supervisors would, you know...' said Durry.

One of the changes that Durry and the WHO made was to persuade the federal and provincial governments to remove the polio programme from the purview of the health department and place it directly under the head of the district administration. Consequently, these heads were accountable for the success of the programme. The WHO then insisted that a method be set up for vaccinators to be paid directly by the polio programme, into their bank accounts. 'All the people doing stuff in the middle were out.'

These changes to the administrative system and growing international pressure brought about a gradual improvement in the immunisation programme. So too did greater public pressure from within Pakistan to eradicate polio quickly so that Pakistan would not continue to suffer the indignity of being the last country in the world to eradicate the disease. But there was a price to be paid in terms of the demands that repeated polio vaccination campaigns were placing on government officials and vaccinators, which I saw when I sat in on a meeting at the district administration office in Rawalpindi. Rawalpindi, is a sprawling city that adjoins the Pakistani capital Islamabad. It is where the Pakistani army has its headquarters and by the country's standards, it is a well-run and well-resourced city.

It was the morning of a two-day vaccination campaign and the meeting was held in a long, dark, conference room at the office of the head of the local health department, Dr Zafar Iqbal Gondal. Rawalpindi was one of the major transit points for refugees streaming out of the frontier regions to escape the fighting between the army and the Taliban. The aim of the day's campaign was to immunise as many of the refugee children coming into the city, while also continuing to vaccinate local children and keep their immunity high. Though Rawalpindi had not recorded an actual case of polio for some years, tests of the city's sewage water showed that the virus was present in the city.

Sitting around the table that day were local health department officials, and representatives from the WHO, UNICEF and Rotary, and as the meeting proceeded, it was apparent that the health department was short staffed and overstressed by the need for repeated polio vaccination. There had been twenty campaigns that year already, and since door to door vaccinations were scheduled on weekends, vaccinators either missed their weekly days off, or took a day off during the week, leaving a gap in the health department's functioning. The health department simply did not have enough vaccinators to send out twice a month on day-long to door-to-door campaigns. The campaign that day required sixty-three mobile teams at bus stations and transit points to vaccinate children getting off buses from the border areas. The health department only had enough vaccinators for twenty-six teams that day, which meant a large number of refugee children would not be vaccinated. The shortage of manpower was exacerbated by a lack of Pashto speaking vaccinators. The refugees coming into the city were Pashto speaking, while Rawalpindi is a Punjabi speaking city and the health department did not have enough Pashto speaking employees, 'We need ninety-one language appropriate teams, and we are short forty-nine,' Dr Ehsan, the health department official overseeing polio told the meeting. His boss, Dr Gondal looked around the conference room and said 'I need help from other departments. My health department does not have enough people.' There were officials from other departments sitting around the table, but no one volunteered additional manpower. As the discussion continued, other issues came to the fore. There was a high turnover of staff, perhaps because of the workload, and there was not enough time to train new staff when they came in. Despite all this the mood was upbeat, and Dr Gondal ended the meeting with an exhortation: 'We are behind Nigeria and Afghanistan in this fight. We have to reach each child. Please monitor your child and get good workers.'

Three years later, in 2017, these intense, draining campaigns are still going on, two times a month, in Rawalpindi and many other areas of Pakistan. I begin to understand why eradication campaigns are meant to be short, intense, and time-bound. It is impossible to maintain this pace year after year. Vaccinators get tired, the public gets tired, government departments can no longer afford to tie up so much time and money. When so many people are chasing a single disease, it is to the inevitable neglect of other diseases.

* * *

The polio programme also tried to address two other causes of public disinterest in the polio programme. First, polio eradication was seen as being inspired and driven by the United States and other Western interests, at a time when anti-Western feeling in Pakistan, whether among the poor or the wealthier section of society was running high. Second, polio was seen as a marginal and trivial disease compared to the other health challenges that children in Pakistan faced.

To de-westernize the face of polio eradication, the Pakistan government turned to the Middle East for funds and material support. Loans and grants were taken from the Islamic Development Bank, Saudi Arabia and the UAE for vaccine purchases as well as to meet the other costs of the programme. 'Instead of being a western-driven programme, it has become an Islamic-driven programme,' remarked Dr Azra Pechucho, who led Pakistan's polio efforts during the earlier Pakistan People's Party regime. 'This was a delinking of the programme from being an UN driven, western-driven one, to allay fears that the west had a premeditated or vested interest in saying that polio had been eradicated.'[29]

The UAE, which hosts a large population of Pakistanis, was roped in as a key funder of the polio programme in Pakistan, through a relationship that Bill Gates had built with the crown prince of Abu Dhabi, Mohammed bin Zayed. Gates and the Abu Dhabi Crown Prince had formed a partnership to fund the purchase of childhood vaccines for children in Pakistan in 2011. This was used for polio immunisation in the frontier areas of Pakistan, marketed as the UAE Pakistan Assistance Programme.

One of the most obvious weakness of the polio programme was that it dealt with only a single disease. An ambitious attempt was made to re-brand the polio programme, and in fact make it about everything but polio, in one of Pakistan's frontier provinces, Khyber Pakhtunkhwa.

Khyber Pakhtunkhwa was the home province of the cricketer turned politician Imran Khan, and the party he had founded, the Pakistan Tehreek-e-Insaaf, ruled the provincial government. Durry, working with a communication consultant Babar Atta who was close to Imran Khan, devised a strategy whereby the provincial government would launch a new health scheme called Sehat ka Insaaf, which would target not just polio but a host of other childhood diseases. It was also branded as an initiative by Imran Khan, that had nothing to do with the polio programme. In fact, every effort was made to completely distance Sehat ka Insaaf from the polio programme. 'This programme is being run by local people in accordance with local traditions,' a spokesman for Sehat ka Insaaf was quoted as saying.[30] Imran Khan had carved for himself an anti-Western image, which in turn helped the polio campaign shed its "western" image.

There was a little sleight of hand involved in all of this. This was still very much a WHO planned polio campaign, except that the WHO and its other international partners stayed well behind the scenes. Even though it was branded as a campaign to protect against nine diseases, the only vaccine distributed by the immunisation that went door-to-door was polio. For the other vaccines that had been promised, families were given coupons to go to their nearest public clinic or hospital, and their children immunised, which they could do anyway under the regular childhood immunisation programme.

But this sleight of hand was apparently enough for people to be convinced that this was a new scheme, and a record number of children were immunised, and more important there was a sharp fall in the number of cases of polio in the province. It was not just re-branding. There was also a much smarter security plan than had been used in other parts of the countries. Since most of the shooting of polio vaccinators had been carried out by men on motorcycles, there was a ban on motorcycles in areas where the campaign was being conducted. Whole localities were cordoned off by security forces on campaign days. The polio programme also used a new strategy of day-long rather than the more traditional three day long campaigns.

Khyber Pakhtunkhwa, and its capital city Peshawar was a nodal point for polio epidemiology in Pakistan. If the routes along which the poliovirus circulated in Pakistan were mapped out, the tribal regions of North and South Waziristan—where vaccination had been banned by the Taliban, and where the poliovirus transmitted in the population unhindered—would appear like a beating heart, pumping out large quantities of polio cases as well as the virus. The virus would then be taken by people fleeing the fighting to Peshawar, the largest and most prominent city of the Pashtu people in Pakistan, where refugees from the war often had family members and fellow clansmen to take shelter with. From Peshawar, the virus would travel to other parts of the country, particularly Rawalpindi and Islamabad, as well as further south to Karachi. Karachi, was like a second heart from where the virus would be pumped to other parts of the country. The outlying suburbs of Karachi had large, long settled Pashtu populations, who offered shelter to refugees from the fighting in the border areas. The shooting of vaccinators in 2012 brought a temporary suspension in polio vaccination, allowing the virus to replicate and transmit unchecked. Travellers leaving Karachi would then carry the virus back to the frontier areas and the neighbouring province of Baluchistan.

POLIO

From a high of thirty cases in 2014, Karachi had come down to zero cases of polio in the first half of 2017. Part of the reason was the improved security that the Sindh government and paramilitary forces provided for vaccinators. But perhaps a more important reason was a rebranding in Karachi as well of the polio programme into a general health programme, through health camps that provided not only polio drops and other medicines for children, but also treated mothers for their various ailments.

In early 2015, I visited one of the first such health camps in Karachi. A few months earlier, I had been part of an armed procession of vaccinators knocking on doors and trying to persuade distrustful parents to get their children vaccinated. This time around, a school had been converted into a makeshift health care centre, run by local doctors and volunteers from the Aga Khan University medical school in Karachi. A steady stream of women with their children waited patiently to see the doctors, who vaccinated the children against polio, but spent an equal amount of time listening to the mothers' problems, and dispensing drugs for minor ailments. There were a few policemen outside the compound, but their presence was largely unnecessary. The health camp was responding to something the community needed, and not even the Taliban dared intervene.

EPILOGUE

The Long Road to Zero

As 2018 dawned, it was hard to tell whether polio's odyssey of eradication was about to reach journey's end or whether the virus and its vaccine-derived cousins would continue to evade the strenuous, but increasingly fatigue-ridden, efforts of the Global Polio Eradication Initiative to pump as much vaccine into as many children as many times as possible in the districts of Pakistan and Afghanistan where it was still actively circulating. This was besides the challenge of rushing to put down outbreaks in countries that had been thought to be polio-free.

The polio eradication campaign was as usual unfailingly optimistic in public: only seventeen cases had been reported in the year, all in Pakistan and Afghanistan. One more year of vaccination campaigns, and the virus could well be stamped out. '2018 will bring the world's best opportunity yet to end the disease,' the polio Global Polio Eradication Initiative wrote in a year-end message.[1]

This was not the first time the polio eradication campaign had declared the world was on the verge of eradicating polio. For much of the last two decades, this had been the campaign's consistent theme. The number of cases of polio had decreased by 99.9 per cent since 1988 when the eradication campaign was launched and 16 million children had been saved from paralysis. All that needed to be done was to wipe out the poliovirus from its last few strongholds.

But it was more complex than that. In 2017, while cases of polio caused by wild poliovirus were indeed at an all-time low, cases of vaccine-derived polio had shot up due to outbreaks in Syria and the

Democratic Republic of Congo. Both outbreaks showed how easy it was for both the wild poliovirus as well as vaccine-derived polioviruses to spread undetected in conflict ridden parts of the world. And they also showed the surprising resilience of vaccine-derived polio strains.

More than seventy cases of vaccine-derived polio in Syria occurred in 2017, in conditions that were almost tailor-made for the Sabin vaccine virus to mutate and spread. After Islamic State forces had occupied parts of eastern Syria the routine vaccination of children became an early casualty of the war. Polio vaccine had only rarely reached children from around 2012. The steady build-up in numbers of susceptible children allowed the vaccine virus to spread in the community, acquiring mutations and becoming increasingly lethal as it spread.

More than seventy of these cases were in the eastern governorate of Deir er-Zor, which until November had been under the control of ISIS and had been the scene of battles between the Syrian army and ISIS. The polio campaign had made heroic efforts to vaccinate children in Deir er-Zor and Raqqa, the Islamic State's de facto capital city, until November 2017, when Kurdish forces took the city. Unlike Nigeria and Pakistan, demand for vaccines from parents were high in Syria and elsewhere in the Middle East: the problem was negotiating with multiple armed groups, including the Syrian army, for access to these areas.

The most serious cause for worry though was the fact that the Syrian outbreak had been caused by a Type 2 vaccine-derived poliovirus. The Type 2 Sabin vaccine was known to be responsible for the majority of outbreaks of vaccine-derived polio. A WHO advisory group on vaccines, the SAGE group, had insisted it be withdrawn from use, especially since the natural Type 2 virus it was meant to protect against had been extinct since 1999. The Type 2 vaccine was therefore withdrawn globally in May 2016. Genetic analysis of the vaccine-derived viruses in Syria showed they had been circulating for well over a year among children (and probably adults as well).

The polio campaign's plan had been to introduce one or two doses of Salk type inactivated polio vaccine (IPV) to protect children against any residual Type 2 vaccine viruses. But poor planning and a reluctance on the part of manufacturers to commit to producing large quantities of vaccine for which they were not sure how much demand there would be led to critical shortages of IPV. The only way to stamp out cases of vaccine-derived Type 2 virus was to go back to using Type 2 OPV to immunise children in Syria. The Type 2 OPV was extremely effective in stamping out cases of vaccine-derived polio, but its extensive use reintroduced the vaccine virus into the environment. This created conditions for new outbreaks of vaccine-derived polio. The polio campaign was fighting fire with fire. Privately among the polio campaign partners, there was nervousness about this strategy, which could well be laying the foundation for cases of vaccine-derived polio a year or two down the road.

The eruption of vaccine-derived polio cases in the Democratic Republic of Congo (DRC) in 2017 illustrated another set of problems that were common to many of the poorest countries in the world. The DRC is the largest country by area in sub-Saharan Africa, and also among the poorest and most populated. Though it had been officially declared polio-free, health services were non-existent in the more far flung parts of the country. There were villages in the south-eastern parts of the countries that did not appear on maps, and others that vaccination teams find difficult to reach because of rough terrain. Also, for the DRC government, polio was little more than a minor irritant compared to a more urgent outbreak of ebola the same year. The conditions that led to a vaccine-derived Type 2 poliovirus in the Congo were similar to those that existed in other poor countries. These included an absence of wild poliovirus combined with low rates of vaccination coverage that left children vulnerable to polio, either from the natural virus, or from a vaccine-derived virus. Also, like many other poor and conflict-ridden countries the network of doctors, health care workers and community workers that were supposed to detect and report potential cases of polio, was extremely weak. This allowed the virus to circulate undetected for fairly long periods of time.

Despite these outbreaks in supposedly polio-free countries, the polio eradication campaign concentrated its efforts on two countries where the polio was still endemic. These were Pakistan and Afghanistan, where—along with Nigeria—polio transmission was thought to have been interrupted but had not been.

In each of these countries, the picture was mixed. In Pakistan, the number of cases were the lowest they had ever been, but samples of sewage water showed that the virus was still circulating in different parts of the country. The virus was also finding new niches in which to embed in Pakistan. It was consistently turning up in sewage samples in Islamabad, where the government had its seat, and its twin city Rawalpindi, where the military is headquartered, showing that the virus was circulating in both these cities. After a long battle, the polio campaign had cleared Karachi of poliovirus in 2016, but by 2017 it had returned, brought back to the city by travellers from other infected parts of the country as well as Afghanistan. Balochistan, a province bordering Afghanistan had emerged as a hot spot for poliovirus transmission. This was particularly in the district of Killa Abdullah in the northwest of the province, home of the one of the busiest crossing points between Pakistan and Afghanistan.

In Afghanistan the southern provinces of Kandahar and Helmand, where the Taliban is battling for control, have provided ideal terrain for the poliovirus to embed itself and spread to other parts of the country. The Taliban in Afghanistan (unlike the Pakistan Taliban) have said they do not object to polio vaccination, but insist that all vaccinators should be hired from areas they control to ensure they are not spies. They have also insisted that vaccinators are not accompanied by Afghan government security forces. But access is still difficult, often based on the whims of local commanders. Even when there is access, there is the perennial problem of convincing a sceptical population of the need for repeated vaccination for a disease that they were barely aware of. As elsewhere in the world, of all the diseases that afflicted the children of Afghanistan, polio was one of the rarest. Yet again it was hard to convince a suspicious population of the need to give so much attention to a single disease when other more pressing health issues were ignored.

While the Taliban in Afghanistan allowed polio immunisation, provided their terms were met, Boko Haram in Nigeria had made large parts of the northern Nigerian state of Borno inaccessible. This meant no vaccination or disease surveillance was possible. Today between 150,000 to 200,000 children remain out of reach of the health services, and there is no way to know whether the poliovirus circulates among them or not. Nigeria had been thought to be polio-free after not reporting a single case for two years between 2014 and 2016. In August 2016, two children were found in Borno state with polio, and genetic analysis established the poliovirus had been transmitting in the state all the while that Nigeria had been thought to be polio-free. Polio in northern Nigeria also brought the danger that the virus had spread to the equally inaccessible and inhospitable border areas of Chad and Nigeria, including remote populations living around Lake Chad, and on islands in the lake.

As the polio eradication campaign continued to chase the poliovirus, it was also running out of time and money. Its most recent timeline for eradication had hoped for eradication to be achieved by 2016. As 2017 ended with the poliovirus still in circulation, it was clear that the next best hope was to reach the magic figure of zero cases of polio by the end of 2018. If that did happen, it would take another three years of waiting and searching for polio cases across the world, whether from wild or vaccine-derived poliovirus, before a global certification commission could certify that polio was eradicated.

But the story would still not end. The risks of the poliovirus still existing in some corner of the world undetected, from where it could be reintroduced to other parts of the world by travellers and cause new epidemics, would remain. Therefore countries would have to continue to vaccinate children against polio, using IPV for at least another ten years. Disease surveillance systems would have to be at work across the world to detect and respond quickly to any outbreak of polio. When the countries of the world voted in 1988 to eradicate polio by 2000, none of this was foreseen. The assumption at the time was that once polio had been eradicated, vaccination against polio could stop within a few years at the most. But experience had shown that it was possible for the poliovirus to transmit for several years undetected, especially since most polio infections are symptomless. In Borno state in Nigeria for example, both wild polio as well as vaccine-derived polioviruses had spread undetected for two years.

At the time of writing, there is also a limit to how long even organisations as invested in polio eradication as the Bill and Melinda Gates Foundation and Rotary will be able to raise funds. The project has dragged on for decades beyond its original deadline. The polio eradication campaigns spends US$1 billion a year now, largely in Afghanistan, Pakistan, Nigeria, and countries where polio has re-appeared, or is in danger of re-appearing. Every additional year that passes without eradication being achieved, makes it harder to justify spending this amount on containing a single disease that is confined to a handful of pockets of the world.

The word most used to describe the mood in the polio eradication campaign is fatigue. After more than two decades of struggle against a virus that seems to keep popping up when it is expected to disappear, it appears the polio eradication campaign is running short of ideas. As a report by the polio campaign's Independent Monitoring Board put it 'Some observers have remarked that the Polio Programme has run out of ideas at risk of coming to a stalemate in its battle with the poliovirus. Many have remarked...that a pervasive sense of fatigue and low spirit seems to be permeating the GPEI. A small number of leaders reflected privately on whether eradication is even possible and whether even if it has been achieved, the Polio Programme will know that it has been done.'[2]

The smallpox eradication campaign too went through similar crises of confidence before the disease was finally stamped out, so it could well be that polio eradicators will finally get the better of the virus they have been chasing these last few decades. As D A Henderson, a key figure in the smallpox eradication campaign declared once it was all over 'It was only by the grace of God that that events happened as they did and allowed execution of the Smallpox Eradication Programme.'[3]

The long battle between the polio eradication campaign and the poliovirus could well end in victory. When that happens, it will be hailed as a major triumph not only in the history of public health, but human history as well. It would mark only the second time that a disease-causing microbe has been rendered extinct through an organised campaign. But it will be an uncertain victory. It will take at least another decade for the world to be really sure that the poliovirus is indeed extinct. It will be a victory that will be overshadowed by the fact that humans are rapidly acquiring the ability to synthesise viruses, including as Eckard Wimmer has shown, the poliovirus. Therefore it may not be wise to stop vaccinating against polio.

It will be a victory marked by great acts of sacrifice including that of at least 100 vaccinators and policemen assassinated by the Taliban in Pakistan and Boko Haram in Nigeria. It will be a victory marked by some of the finest technical achievements in public health in terms of disease surveillance, outbreak response, and the ability to reach vaccines to children in the most difficult of conditions. But it is also a victory marked by ethical dilemmas, chiefly caused by the use of a vaccine that was cheap, easily deliverable, but also caused paralysis in some who received it.

The original decision by World Health Assembly to eradicate polio was, as we have seen, taken almost on a whim, with no consideration of how much it would cost, and the difficulties that might lie ahead. A review was commissioned by the WHO of the polio programme in 2001. It declared that for future programmes, 'it would be desirable for the WHO to ensure that the technical, managerial, and resource aspects of an initiative have been examined carefully before a resolution is sought from the Health Assembly.'[4]

The polio eradication partners were unlikely to have embarked on the project had they known how long, difficult and costly it was going to turn out to be.

The polio campaign, even if successful, will not resolve the long-standing debate about whether so called vertical programmes, targeting a single disease, do more to contribute to health than 'horizontal programmes' that strengthen health systems and target multiple diseases. The world has already spent close to US$15 billion on targeting a single disease. Would this money have had a bigger impact on the health of children if it had been spent on broader vaccination programmes? The WHO and UNICEF are also partners in a Global Immunisation Vision and Strategy that aims to reduce the number of deaths of children under the age of five by protecting them through vaccination against fourteen diseases, including polio. If 90 per cent of the world's children were immunised against these diseases, it is estimated that two million deaths a year of children under five could be prevented. A financial analysis in 2008 estimated that this would cost about US$35 billion for seventy-two of the world's poorest countries to achieve this goal over a nine-year period. If the money spent by the polio eradication campaign had gone into broader vaccine programmes (including polio vaccination), perhaps the world's children would be better off today.

As we have seen, the polio eradication campaign also shone a stark light on the huge gap between local health needs and global health programmes. It was difficult (and still is) for people in poor countries facing multiple health needs to understand why a disease that they did not consider to be important, was given such priority. This was to the extent that people were threatened with jail in Pakistan and Nigeria for refusing to vaccinate their children. If there is a lesson from this for future global programmes, it is that their task would be far easier if they were more responsive to the needs of the people that they were supposed to serve, rather than the well-meaning donors funding their projects.

NOTES

PROLOGUE

1. Soper, F. L. (1962), *The Yellow Fever Lecture Notes*, Harvard, 1962, US National Library of Medicine.
2. Taylor, C. E., Cutts, F. and Taylor M. E. (1997), 'Ethical Dilemmas in Current Planning for Polio Eradication', *American Journal of Public Health*, 87(6).
3. Dybul, M., Piot, P., and Frenk, J (2012), 'Reshaping Global Health', *Policy Review*, Stanford, CA: Hoover Institution.
4. Platt, L., Estivariz, C. and Sutter, R. W. (2014), 'Vaccine-Associated Paralytic Poliomyelitis: A Review of the Epidemiology and Estimation of the Global Burden', *Journal of Infectious Diseases*, (Suppl 1).
5. Aylward, B., 'How we'll stop polio for good', TED Talk, https://www.ted.com/talks/bruce_aylward_how_we_ll_stop_polio.
6. Block, S. M. (2002), 'A Not So Cheap Stunt', *Science*, 297.

1. THE SHADOWY WORLD OF THE POLIOVIRUS

1. Hippocrates (1973), *Hippocratic Writings* Trans. Chadwick, J. and Mann, W. N., London: Penguin.
2. Smallman-Raynor, M. R. and Cliff, A. D. (2006). *Poliomyelitis: A World Geography: Emergence to Eradication*, Oxford: Oxford University Press.
3. Axelsson, P. (2009), '"Do Not Eat Those Apples; They've been on the Ground!": Polio Epidemics and Preventive Measures, Sweden 1880s–1940s', *Ascelpio, Revista de Historia de la Medicinia y de la Ciencia*.
4. Ibid.
5. Paul, J. R. (1971), *A History of Poliomyelitis*, New Haven, CT: Yale University Press.
6. Horstmann, D. M. (1985), *The Poliomyelitis Story: A Scientific Hegira*, *The Yale Journal of Biology and Medicine*, 58, 79–90.

7. Crawford, D. H. (2011), *Viruses: A Very Short Introduction*, Oxford: Oxford University Press.
8. Racaniello, V. R. (2006), 'One hundred years of poliovirus pathogenesis', *Virology*, 344.
9. McNeill, W. H. (1976), *Plagues and Peoples*, New York: Anchor Books.
10. Smallman-Raynor, M. R. and Cliff, A. D. (2006), *Poliomyelitis. A World Geography: Emergence to Eradication*, Oxford: Oxford University Press.
11. McNeill, *Plagues and Peoples*.

2. THE PRESIDENT AND THE POLIOVIRUS

1. Goldman, A. S. et al (2016), 'Franklin Delano Roosevelt's (FDR's) (1882–1945) 1921 neurological disease revisited; the most likely diagnosis remains Guillaume–Barré syndrome', *Journal of Medical Biography*, 24(4), 452–459.
2. Ditunno, J. F., Jr Becker, B. E., and Herbison, G. J. (2016), *Franklin Delano Roosevelt: The Diagnosis of Poliomyelitis Revisited*, PM&R. 8(9): p. 883–893.
3. Fairchild, A. L. (2001), 'The Polio Narratives: Dialogues with FDR', *Bulletin of the History of Medicine*, 75(3), 488–534.
4. Oshinsky, D. M. (2005), *Polio: An American Story*, New York: Oxford University Press.
5. Smith, J. S. (1990), *Patenting the Sun: Polio and the Salk Vaccine*, New York: W. Morrow, 413.
6. Ibid.
7. Wilson, D. J. (1998), 'A Crippling Fear: Experiencing Polio in the Era of FDR', *Bulletin of the History of Medicine*, 72(3), 464–495.
8. Oshinsky, *Polio: An American Story*, viii, 342, 16 p of plates.
9. Ibid.
10. Smith, J. E. (2007), *FDR*, New York: Random House, 858.
11. Oshinsky, *Polio: An American Story*.
12. Nathanson, N. and Kew, O. M. (2010), 'From Emergence to Eradication: The Epidemiology of Polio Deconstructed', *American Journal of Epidemiology*, 172(11).
13. Wilson, D. J. (2005), *Living With Polio: The Epidemic and its Survivors*, Chicago, IL: University of Chicago Press.
14. Gould, T. (1995), *A Summer Plague: Polio and its Survivors*, New Haven, CT: Yale University Press.
15. Shiffman, J., Beer, T. and Wu, Y. (2002), 'The Emergence of Global Disease Control Priorities', *Health Policy and Planning*, 17(3), 225–234. doi:10.1093/heapol/17.3.225
16. Cook, S. G. (2013), 'Rotary and the Gift of a Polio-Free World', *Volume 1: Making the Promise*, Evanston, IL: Rotary International.

3. THE SALK VACCINE: ENDING THE TERROR OF POLIO

1. Paul, J R (1971), *A History of Poliomyelitis*, New Haven and London: Yale University Press.
2. Ibid.
3. Leake, J P (1935), 'Poliomyelitis following vaccination against this disease', *Journal of the American Medical Association*.
4. Oshinsky, D M (2005), *Polio: An American Story*, New York: Oxford University Press. viii, 342 p, 16 p of plates.
5. Paul, *A History of Poliomyelitis*.
6. Ibid.
7. DeCroes, Jacobs, C (2015), *Jonas Salk: A Life*, New York: Oxford University Press.
8. Paul, *A History of Poliomyelitis*.
9. Eggers, H J (1999), 'Milestones in Early Poliomyelitis Research (1840 to 1949)', *Journal of Virology*, 73(6): p. 4533–4535.
10. Troan, J (2000), *Passport to Adventure: Memoirs of a Twentieth Century News Correspondent and Science Writer*, John Troan.
11. Salk, J E (1954), 'Formaldehyde Treatment and Safety Testing of Experimental Poliomyelitis Vaccines', *American Journal of Public Health*, 44(5).
12. Ibid.
13. DeCroes, *Jonas Salk: A Life*.
14. Oshinsky, *Polio: An American Story*, viii, 342, 16 p of plates.
15. Ibid.
16. Salk, J E, et al. (1954), 'Studies in Human Subjects on Active Immunisation Against Poliomyelitis', *American Journal of Public Health*, 44.
17. DeCroes, Jacobs, C (2015), *Jonas Salk: A Life*, New York: Oxford University Press.
18. Paul, *A History of Poliomyelitis*.
19. DeCroes, *Jonas Salk: A Life*.

4. A TOOL FOR ERADICATION: ALBERT SABIN AND THE ORAL POLIO VACCINE

1. Hailey, F (1954), 'Doctor Criticizes Polio Vaccine Use', *The New York Times*.
2. Oshinsky, D M (2005), *Polio: An American Story*, New York: Oxford University Press. viii, 342, 16 p of plates.
3. Ibid.
4. Sabin A.B. and Korporwski H., Correspondence. (1957) Hauck Centre for the Albert B. Sabin Archives, Cinncinna.

5. Koprowski, H. and Sabin A.B. Correspondence. (1958) Hauck Centre for the Albert B Sabin Archives, Cincinnati.
6. Sabin A.B. and Koprowski, H. Correspondence. (1958) Hauk Centre for the Albert B Sabin Archives, Cinncinnati.
7. Fox, M (2013), 'Hilary Koprowski, Who Developed First Live-Virus Polio Vaccine, Dies at 96', in *New York Times*: http://www.nytimes.com/2013/04/21/us/hilary-koprowski-developed-live-virus-polio-vaccine-dies-at-96.html.
8. Sabin, A B, Transcript of an interview of Albert B Sabin conducted by Saul Benison, May 15 1976, Benison, S, Editor, Hauk Centre for the Albert B Sabin Archives: Cincinnati.
9. Racaniello, V R (2012), personal interview.
10. Sabin, A B, Transcript of an interview of Albert B Sabin conducted by Saul Benison 23 May 1976, Benison, S, Editor. The Hauk Centre for the Albert B, Sabin Archives: Cincinnati.
11. Ibid.
12. Ibid.
13. Ibid.
14. Sabin, A B, Transcript of an interview of Albert Sabin conducted by Saul Benison June 3 1976, Benison, S, Editor 1976, The Hauk Center for the Albert B Sabin Archives: Cincinnati.
15. Ibid.
16. Ibid.
17. Ibid.
18. Horstmann, D. M. (1991), 'The Sabin Live Poliovirus Vaccination Trials in the USSR', 1959, *Yale Journal of Biology and Medicine*, 64.
19. Sabin, A. B. (1960), 'Live Orally Given Poliovirus Vaccine. Effects of Rapid Mass Immunisation on Population Under Conditions of Massive Enteric Infection With Other Viruses', *The Journal of the American Medical Association*, 173(14).
20. Kaplan, M. (1961), 'Salk Challenges AMA Stand; Delegates Back Sabin Vaccine', in *The New York Times*.
21. Oshinsky, *Polio: An American Story*.
22. Dick, G. W. A. and Dane, D. S. (1959), 'The Evaluation of Live Poliovirus Vaccines', Paper presented at the Live Poliovirus Vaccines Papers Presented and Discussions Held at the First Live International Conference on Live Poliovirus, Washington, DC.
23. Best, E. W. R. and Rhodes, A. J. (1963), 'Live Oral Poliovirus Vaccine in Canada', *Canadian Journal of Public Health*, 54(12).
24. Special Advisory Committee on Oral Poliomyelitis Vaccines, 'Oral Poliomyelitis Vaccines', *Journal of the American Medical Association*, 1964, 190(1).

25. Sabin, A. B. (1964), 'Commentary on Report on Oral Poliomyelitis Vaccines', *Journal of the American Medical Association*, 190(1).
26. Sabin, A. B. (1976), Transcript of an interview of Dr Albert B Sabin by Saul Benison, 4 July 1976, Benison, S. ed. 1976, The Hauk Center for the Albert B Sabin Archives: Cincinnati.
27. Special Advisory Committee on Oral Poliomyelitis Vaccines, 'Oral Poliomyelitis Vaccines', *Journal of the American Medical Association*, 1964, 190(1).
28. IMB. (2010–). Reports of the Independent Monitoring Board of the Global Polio Eradication Initiative Institute of Medicine. (1996). 'Options for Poliomyelitis Vaccination in the United States': Workshop Summary, Washington, DC.
29. Ibid.
30. Platt, L., Estivariz, C. and Sutter, R. W. (2014), 'Vaccine-Associated Paralytic Poliomyelitis: A Review of the Epidemiology and Estimation of the Global Burden', *Journal of Infectious Diseases*, (Suppl 1).
31. Racaniello, V. R. (2012), personal interview.

5. A COALITION OF THE WILLING: THE BIRTH OF THE GLOBAL POLIO ERADICATION INITIATIVE

1. Fenner, F. (1982), 'Global Eradication of Smallpox' (with discussion), *Reviews of Infectious Diseases*, 4(5).
2. Ibid.
3. 'Eradication, Elimination and Control: Which Disease Next?', *Reviews of Infectious Diseases*, 1982, 4(5).
4. 'Conclusions and Recommendations', *Reviews of Infectious Diseases*, 1982, 4(5).
5. Fenner, F. (1982), 'Global Eradication of Smallpox' (with discussion), *Reviews of Infectious Diseases*, 4(5).
6. John, T. J., (1984), 'Poliomyelitis in India: Prospects and Problems of Control', *Reviews of Infectious Diseases*, 6 Supp. 2.
7. Robbins, F. C. (1984), 'Summary and Recommendations,' *Reviews of Infectious Diseases*, 6 Supp. 2.
8. De Quadros, C., 'The Whole is Greater: How Polio Was Eradicated from the Western Hemisphere', in Pelman D. and Roy A. eds, *The Practice of International Health: A Case-Based Orientation*, Oxford: Oxford University Press.
9. Pandak, C Personal Interview 2017.
10. Sever, J., Author, Personal Interview, 2014.
11. Cook, S. G. (2013), 'Rotary and the Gift of a Polio-Free World', *Volume 1: Making the Promise*, Evanston, IL: Rotary International.

12. Ibid.
13. Ibid.
14. Ibid.
15. Pigman, H. A. (2005), *Conquering Polio: A Brief History of PolioPlus, Rotary's Role in a Global Program to Eradicate the World's Greatest Crippling Disease*, Evanston, IL: Rotary International.
16. WHO (2008), 'The Third Ten Years of the World Health Organisation', Geneva: World Health Organisation.
17. Virchow, R. (1848), Report on the Typhus Epidemic in Upper Silesia (English Translation), *Social Medicine*, 1(1).
18. Mahler, H. (2008), 'Primary health care comes full circle. An interview with Dr Halfdan Mahler', *Bulletin of the World Health Organisation*, http://www.who.int/bulletin/volumes/86/10/08–041008/en/
19. De Quadros, C., Personal Interview 2013.
20. De Quadros, C., Personal Interview, 2013.
21. Muraskin, W. (2012), *Polio Eradication and its Discontents: A Historian's Journey Through an International Public Health (Un)Civil War*, Hyderabad: Orient Blackswan.

6. ERADICATING POLIOMYELITIS FROM SPACESHIP EARTH

1. Mahler, H. (1988), 'World Health 2000 and Beyond', Paper presented at the 41st World Health Assembly, Geneva.
2. Mahler, H. Address on the Occasion of the Celebration of the Fortieth Anniversary of WHO and Tenth Anniversary of the Declaration of Alma-Ata During the Forty-First World Health Assembly. In *Forty-first World Heath Assembly*, 1988, Geneva: World Health Organisation.
3. De Quadros, C., Personal Interview, 2013.
4. WHO (1988), 'Forty-First World Health Assembly Verbatim Records of Plenary Meetings Records of Committees', at the Forty-First World Health Assembly, Geneva.

7. A HASTY DECISION AND A SLOW START

1. De Quadros, C., Personal Interview, 2013.
2. Henderson, R. (2016), 'Oral History Rafe Henderson' in Torghele, K. ed., 'David J Sencer CDC Museum, Global Health Chronicles', https://www.globalhealthchronicles.org/items/show/6477
3. WHO (1989), 'World Health Organisation Executive Board Eighty-Second Session Resolutions and Decisions Summary Records'.
4. WHO (1989), 'Global Poliomyelitis Eradication by the Year 2000 Plan of Action', Retrieved from Geneva.
5. Pigman, H. A. (2005), *Conquering Polio: A Brief History of PolioPlus*,

Rotary's Role in a Global Program to Eradicate the World's Greatest Crippling Disease, Evanston, IL: Rotary International.

6. Cook, S. G. (2013), 'Rotary and the Gift of a Polio-Free World', *Volume 1: Making the Promise*, Evanston, IL: Rotary International.

7. Muraskin, W. (2012), *Polio Eradication and its Discontents: A Historian's Journey Through an International Public Health (Un)Civil War*, Hyderabad: Orient Blackswan.

8. World Health Organization, Geneva (1990), 'Eradication of Polio-myelitis. Report of the Third Consultation', Retrieved from Geneva.

9. Sutter, R. W. et al (1991), 'Outbreak of paralytic poliomyelitis in Oman: evidence for widespread transmission among fully vaccinated children', *Lancet*, 338(8769), 715–20.

8. IN THE DOLDRUMS

1. Arita, I., Nakane, M. and Fenner, F. (2006), 'Public health: Is polio eradication realistic?', *Science*, 312(5775), 852–854. doi:10.1126/science.1124959

2. Chan, M. (2007), World Health Organisation, Geneva.

3. Pandak, C., Personal Interview, 2017.

4. Gates, B., (2016), 'Philanthropist Bill Gates talks public health, bio-tech, and the race for the White House', in Branswell, H. and Berke, R., eds. Statnews, 17 June 2016.

5. Berhane, Y., 'Has routine Immunisation in Africa become endangered?', *Lancet Infectious Diseases*, 2009, 9.

6. Ibid.

7. Donaldson, L., 'Meeting the challenges of Global Polio Eradication-Luncheon Keynote', 2015, CSIS Georgetown.

8. Heymann, D. Personal interview. 2017.

9. Ibid.

10. Ibid.

11. Pandak, C., Personal Interview, 2017.

9. ROGUE VACCINES AND ROGUE VIRUSES

1. Kew, O. M. et al (2005), 'Vaccine-derived polioviruses and the endgame strategy for global polio eradication', *Annual Review of Microbiology*, 59, 587–635.

2. Kew, O., Personal Interview, 2017.

3. Ibid.

4. Ibid.

5. WHO (2017), 'What is vaccine-derived polio?', retrieved from http://www.who.int/features/qa/64/en/

6. Duintjer Tebbens, R. J., Pallansch, M. A., Cochi, S. L., Wassilak, S. G., Linkins, J., Sutter, R. W., Thompson, K. M. (2010), 'Economic analysis of the global polio eradication initiative', *Vaccine*, 29(2), 334–343. doi:10.1016/j.vaccine.2010.10.026

7. Dove, A. W. and Racaniello, V. R. (1997), 'The Polio Eradication Effort: Should Vaccine Eradication Be Next?', Science, 277(5327), 779–780. doi:10.1126/science.277.5327.779

8. John, T. J. (2000), 'The Final Stages of The Global Eradication of Polio', *The New England Journal of Medicine*, 343(11).

9. IMB. (2010–). Reports of the Independent Monitoring Board of the Global Polio Eradication Initiative Institute of Medicine. (1996). 'Options for Poliomyelitis Vaccination in the United States': Workshop Summary, Washington, DC.

10. Muraskin, W. (2012), *Polio Eradication and its Discontents: A Historian's Journey Through an International Public Health (Un)Civil War*, Hyderabad: Orient Blackswan.

11. Ibid.

12. John, J., Personal Interview, 2016.

13. Grassly, N. C., Fraser, C., Wenger, J., Deshpande, J. M., Sutter, R. W., Heymann, D. L. and Aylward, R. B. (2006), 'New Strategies for the Elimination of Polio from India', Science, 314(5802), 1150–1153. doi:10.1126/science.1130388

14. WHO (2009), 'Second Meeting of the SAGE Working Group on IPV', Retrieved from World Health Organization Geneva. http://www.who. int/immunization/sage/previous/en/index3.html

10. INDIA: A LONG DIRTY WAR

1. Henderson, D. (2009), *Smallpox: The Death of a Disease*, New York: Prometheus Books.

2. Fenner, F., Henderson, D., Arita, I., Jezek, Z. and Ladnyi, I. D. (1988), 'Smallpox and its eradication', Geneva: World Health Organisation.

3. Jafari, H., Personal Interview, 2017.

4. Rao, K. S., Personal Interview, 2017.

5. AIDAN, 'Memorandum on Pulse Polio', 2008.

6. Muraskin, W. (2012), *Polio Eradication and its Discontents: A Historian's Journey Through an International Public Health (Un)Civil War*, Hyderabad: Orient Blackswan.

7. Kapur, D., Personal Interview, 2016.

8. UNICEF, 'A Critical Leap to Polio Eradication in India', UNICEF: New Delhi.

9. WHO (2001), 'Progress towards poliomyelitis eradication South-East Asia. Weekly Epidemiological Record', 34(76).

10. John, J., Personal Interview, 2016.
11. Grassly, N. C., Wenger, J. Durrani, S., Bahl, S., Deshpande, J. M., Sutter, R. W., Aylward, R. B. (2007), 'Protective Efficacy of a Monovalent Oral Type 1 Poliovirus Vaccine: A Case-control Study', *Lancet*, 369(9570), 1356–1362. doi:10.1016/s0140–6736(07)60531-5
12. *The Economist* (2004), 'An Area of Darkness', https://www.economist.com/node/2423102
13. Hussain, R. S., McGarvey, S. T., Shahab, T. and Fruzzetti, L. M. (2012), 'Fatigue and Fear with Shifting Polio Eradication Strategies in India: A Study of Social Resistance to Vaccination', *PLoS ONE*, 7(9), e46274. doi:10.1371/journal.pone.0046274
14. UNICEF, 'A Critical Leap to Polio Eradication in India', UNICEF: New Delhi.
15. EPOS, (2003), 'Understanding Barriers to Polio Eradication in Uttar Pradesh Final Report', EPOS Health Consultants India Pvt. Ltd: New Delhi.
16. UNICEF, 'A Critical Leap to Polio Eradication in India'.
17. Ibid.
18. Chaturvedi, G. (2008), *The Vital Drop: Communication for Polio Eradication in India*, Thousand Oaks, CA: SAGE Publications.
19. Jafari, H., Personal Interview, 2017.

11. TWO CRISES AND A FINAL VICTORY

1. Cockburn, C. (1988), 'The Work of the WHO Consultative Group on Poliomyelitis Vaccines', *Bulletin of the World Health Organisation*, 66(2).
2. John, J., Personal Interview, 2016.
3. Ibid.
4. Kapur, D., Personal Interview, 2016.
5. Agarwal, R. K. (2008), 'Polio eradication in India: a tale of science, ethics, dogmas and strategy!', *Indian Pediatrics*, 45(5), 349–51.
6. Cochi, S. L., Personal Interview, 2017.
7. John, J., Personal Interview, 2016.
8. Rao, K. S., Personal Interview, 2017.
9. Muliyil, J. P., Personal Interview, 2017.
10. Retrieved from http://www.iple.in/document/the-107-block-plan
11. Jafari, H., Personal Interview 2017.
12. Ibid.
13. Closser, S., Kelly, C., Parris, T. M. et al (2014), 'The Impact of Polio Eradication on Routine Immunisation and Primary Health Care: A Mixed-Methods Study', *The Journal of Infectious Diseases*, Suppl1.
14. Kohler, K. A., Banerjee, K., Hlady, W. G., Andrus, J. K. and Sutter,

R. W. (2002), 'Vaccine-associated paralytic poliomyelitis in India during 1999: Decreased risk despite massive use of oral polio vaccine', *Bulletin of the World Health Organisation*, 80(3).

15. Kohler, K. A., Banerjee, K. and Sutter, R. W. (2002), 'Further clarity on vaccine-associated paralytic polio in India', *Bulletin of the World Health Organisation*, 80(12).

16. ERC, 'Annual Report 2003–2004, Enterovirus Research Centre, Mumbai', 2004, Indian Council of Medical Research, http://icmr.nic.in/annual/erc/2003–04/r4.pdf

17. Bahl, S., Personal Interview, 2017.

18. IAP, IAP recommendations for AFP surveillance, 2007, http://www.iapindia.org/page.php?id=72

12. PAKISTAN: WHERE THE POLIOVIRUS HID IN BIN LADEN'S SHADOW

1. IMB (2014), 'Report of the Independent Monitoring Board of the Global Polio Eradication Initiative, Ninth Report', May 2014, http://polioeradication.org/wp-content/uploads/2016/07/04E.pdf

2. Ilyas, F. (2012), 'Women saving children from crippling disease fall prey to hostility', *Dawn*, Karachi.

3. Marx, W. (2013), 'Pakistan's Polio War', *Financial Times*, https://www.ft.com/content/fe901856-ce40-11e2-a13e-00144feab7de?mhq5j=e2

4. Walsh, D. and McNeill, D. G. Jr (2012), 'Female Vaccination Workers, Essential in Pakistan, Become Prey', *The New York Times*, http://www.nytimes.com/2012/12/21/world/asia/un-halts-vaccine-work-in-pakistan-after-more-killings.html

5. Rehman, Z. (2012), 'Immobilized', *The Friday Times*, http://www.thefridaytimes.com/beta3/tft/article.php?issue=20121228&page=4

6. Walsh, D. and McNeill, D. G. Jr (2012), 'Female Vaccination Workers, Essential in Pakistan, Become Prey', *The New York Times*, http://www.nytimes.com/2012/12/21/world/asia/un-halts-vaccine-work-in-pakistan-after-more-killings.html

7. Yusufzai, A. (2007), 'Impotence Fears Hit Polio Drive', BBC, http://news.bbc.co.uk/2/hi/south_asia/6299325.stm

8. Khan, K. (2007), 'Exclusive: An Interview with Maulana Fazalullah', ValleySwat, http://www.valleyswat.net/articles/fazalullah_interview.html

9. Yahya, M. (2007), 'Polio vaccines—"no thank you!", barriers to polio eradication in Northern Nigeria', *African Affairs*, 106(423), 185–204.

10. Ghinai, I. et al (2013), 'Listening to the rumours: What the northern Nigeria polio vaccine boycott can tell us ten years on', *Global Public Health*, 8(10).

11. Williams, M. (2012), 'US defence secretary Leon Panetta criticises Pakistan for doctor's sentence', *The Guardian*, https://www.theguardian.com/world/2012/may/27/defence-secretary-leon-panetta-pakistan

12. Nasruminallah (2012), 'No polio drives in N Waziristan unless drone strikes stop: Hafiz Gul Bahadur', *The Express Tribune*, https://tribune.com.pk/story/394714/no-polio-drives-in-n-waziristan-unless-drone-strikes-stop-hafiz-gul-bahadur/

13. The Bureau of Investigative Journalists, Drone Warfare, retrieved from https://www.thebureauinvestigates.com/projects/drone-wa

14. Ibid.

15. Correspondent (2012),'Polio vaccination banned in South Waziristan', *The Express Tribune*, https://tribune.com.pk/story/399274/polio-vaccination-banned-in-south-waziristan/

16. McNeil, D. G. J. (2012), 'CIA Vaccine Ruse May Have Harmed the War on Polio', *The New York Times*, http://www.nytimes.com/2012/07/10/health/cia-vaccine-ruse-in-pakistan-may-have-harmed-polio-fight.html?pagewanted=all

17. Memon, A., Personal Interview, 2014.

18. Abid, N., Personal Interview, 2014.

19. Deans of School of Public Health (2013), 'CIA Vaccination Cover in Pakistan', https://www.jhsph.edu/news/news-releases/2013/klag-CIA-vaccination-cover-pakistan.html

20. Chappell, B. (2014), 'CIA Says It Will No Longer Use Vaccine Programs As Cover', NPR, https://www.npr.org/sections/thetwo-way/2014/05/20/314231260/cia-says-it-will-no-longer-use-vaccine-programs-as-cover

21. Zia, A. S. (2013), 'Pakistan's War on Polio Workers', *The Guardian*, https://www.theguardian.com/commentisfree/2013/jan/03/pakistan-war-polio-workers

22. Ud Din, I., Mumtaz, Z. and Ataullahjan, A. (2012), 'How the Taliban undermined community healthcare in Swat, Pakistan', *British Medical Journal*, 344.

23. Ibid.

24. Memon A, Personal Interview 2014.

25. Bhutta, Z. A. (2014), 'Polio eradication hinges on child health in Pakistan', *Nature*, 511.

26. Yasin, A. and Junaidi, I. (2014), 'Polio certificate for air travellers is a messy affair', *Dawn*, https://www.dawn.com/news/1110267/polio-certificate-for-air-travellers-is-a-messy-affair

27. 'PM Nawaz to deliver a polio free country in six months', *The Express Tribune*, 2014, https://tribune.com.pk/story/786101/pm-nawaz-to-supervise-polio-campaign/

28. Durry, E., Personal Interview, 2014
29. Pehucho, A., Personal Interview, 2015
30. Yusufzai, A. (104), 'Sehat Ka Insaf being extended to entire KP', *Dawn*, https://www.dawn.com/news/1087613

EPILOGUE

1. GPEI (2017), 'Working Toward a Polio-free Future: 2017', *Review*, http://polioeradication.org/news-post/working-toward-a-polio-free-future-2017-in-review/
2. IMB (2017), 'Every Last Hiding Place. 15th Report of the Independent Monitoring Board of the Global Polio Eradication Initiative', http://polioeradication.org/wp-content/uploads/2017/12/polio-eradication-15th-IMB-Report-2017–11.pdf
3. Henderson, D. (1988), 'Eradication: Lessons from the Past', *Bulletin of the World Health Organisation*, 76(Suppl 2), 5.
4. WHO (2001), 'Thematic Evaluations in 2001 Eradication of Poliomyelitis', Report by the Director General Retrieved from Geneva.

SELECT BIBLIOGRAPHY

Arita, I., Nakane, M. and Fenner, F. (2006), 'Public health. Is polio eradication realistic?', *Science*, 312(5775), 852–854. doi:10.1126/science.1124959

Batniji, R. (2008), 'Coordination and accountability in the World Health Assembly', *The Lancet*, 372, 1.

Benison, S. (1974), 'Poliomyelitis and the Rockefeller Institute: Social effects and institutional response', *Journal of the History of Medicine and Allied Sciences*, 29(1), 74–92.

————, Transcripts of Interviews of Albert B Sabin. Hauk Centre for the Albert B Sabin Archives, University of Cincinnati.

Bennett-Jones, O. (2009), *Pakistan: Eye of the Storm*, New Haven, CT: Yale University Press.

Bhattacharya, S. and Dasgupta, R. (2009), 'A Tale of Two Global Health Programs: Smallpox Eradication's Lessons for the Antipolio Campaign in India', *American Journal of Public Health*, 99(7), 1176–1184. doi:10.2105/ajph.2008.135624

Black, K. (1996), *In the Shadow of Polio: A Personal and Social History*, Reading, MA: Addison-Wesley.

Blume, S., and Geesink, I. (2000), 'A Brief History of Polio Vaccines', *Science*, 288(2).

Cáceres, V. M. and Sutter, R. W. (2001), 'Sabin Monovalent Oral Polio Vaccines: Review of Past Experiences and Their Potential Use after Polio Eradication', *Clinical Infectious Diseases*, 33.

Chaturvedi, G. (2008), *The Vital Drop: Communication for Polio Eradication in India*, Thousand Oaks, CA: SAGE Publications.

Chaturvedi, S., Dasgupta, R., Adish, V., Ganguly, K., Rai, K., Sushant, S. et al (2009), 'Deconstructing Social Resistance to Pulse Polio Campaign in Two North Indian Districts', *Indian Pediatrics*, 46(11).

Closser, S. (2010). *Chasing Polio in Pakistan: Why the World's Largest Public Health Initiative Might Fail*, Nashville, TN: Vanderbilt University Press.

SELECT BIBLIOGRAPHY

Closser, S., Kelly, C., Parris, T. M. et al (2014), 'The Impact of Polio Eradication on Routine Immunisation and Primary Health Care: A Mixed-Methods Study', *The Journal of Infectious Diseases*, Supp1.

Cockburn, C. (1988), 'The Work of the WHO Consultative Group on Poliomyelitis Vaccines', *Bulletin of the World Health Organisation*, 66(2).

Cook, S. G. (2013), 'Rotary and the Gift of a Polio-Free World', *Volume 1: Making the Promise*, Evanston, IL: Rotary International.

Crawford, D. H. (2011), *Viruses: A Very Short Introduction*, Oxford: Oxford University Press.

Daniel, T. M. and Robbins, F. C. eds, (2000), *Polio*, Rochester, NY: University of Rochester Press.

De Quadros, C., 'The Whole is Greater: How Polio Was Eradicated from the Western Hemisphere', in Pelman D. and Roy A. eds, *The Practice of International Health: A Case-Based Orientation*, Oxford: Oxford University Press.

DeCroes Jacobs, C. (2015), *Jonas Salk: A Life*, Oxford: Oxford University Press.

Dick, G. W. A. and Dane, D. S. (1959), 'The Evaluation of Live Poliovirus Vaccines', Paper presented at the Live Poliovirus Vaccines Papers Presented and Discussions Held at the First Live International Conference on Live Poliovirus, Washington, DC.

Dove, A. W. and Racaniello, V. R. (1997), 'The Polio Eradication Effort: Should Vaccine Eradication Be Next?', *Science*, 277(5327), 779–780. doi:10.1126/science.277.5327.779

Dowdle, W. R. and Hopkins, D. R. (1998), 'The Eradication of Infectious Diseases: Report of the Dahlem Workshop on the Eradication of Infectious Diseases', Berlin, 16–22 March 1997, Chichester: Wiley.

Duintjer Tebbens, R. J., Pallansch, M. A., Cochi, S. L., Wassilak, S. G., Linkins, J., Sutter, R. W., Thompson, K. M. (2010), 'Economic analysis of the global polio eradication initiative', *Vaccine*, 29(2), 334–343. doi:10.1016/j.vaccine.2010.10.026

Dybul, M., Piot, P., and Frenk, J. (2012), 'Reshaping Global Health', *Policy Review*.

Eggers, H. J. (1999), 'Milestones in Early Poliomyelitis Research (1840 to 1949)', *Journal of Virology*, 73(6), 4533–4535.

Fairchild, A. L. (2001), 'The Polio Narratives: Dialogues with FDR', *Bulletin of the History of Medicine*, 75(3), 488–534.

Fenner, F. (1982), 'Global Eradication of Smallpox' (with discussion), *Reviews of Infectious Diseases*, 4(5).

Fenner, F., Henderson, D., Arita, I., Jezek, Z. and Ladnyi, I. D. (1988), 'Smallpox and its eradication', Geneva: World Health Organisation.

Gallagher, H. G. (1985), *FDR's Splendid Deception* (1st ed.), New York: Dodd, Mead.

SELECT BIBLIOGRAPHY

Gould, T. (1995), *A Summer Plague: Polio and Its Survivors*, New Haven, CT: Yale University Press.

Grassly, N. C. (2013), 'The Final Stages of the Global Eradication of Poliomyelitis', *Philosophical Transactions of the Royal Society B: Biological Sciences*, 368(1623). doi:10.1098/rstb.2012.0140

————, Fraser, C., Wenger, J., Deshpande, J. M., Sutter, R. W., Heymann, D. L. and Aylward, R. B. (2006), 'New Strategies for the Elimination of Polio from India', *Science*, 314(5802), 1150–1153. doi:10.1126/science.1130388

————, Jafari, H., Bahl, S., Durrani, S., Wenger, J., Sutter, R. W. and Aylward, R. B. (2010), 'Asymptomatic Wild-Type Poliovirus Infection in India among Children with Previous Oral Poliovirus Vaccination', *Journal of Infectious Diseases*, 201(10), 1535–1543. doi:10.1086/651952

————, Wenger, J. Durrani, S., Bahl, S., Deshpande, J. M., Sutter, R. W., Aylward, R. B. (2007), 'Protective Efficacy of a Monovalent Oral Type 1 Poliovirus Vaccine: A Case-control Study', *Lancet*, 369(9570), 1356–1362. doi:10.1016/s0140–6736(07)60531–5

Henderson, D. (1988), 'Eradication: Lessons from the Past', *Bulletin of the World Health Organisation*, 76(Suppl 2), 5.

———— (2009), *Smallpox: The Death of a Disease*, New York: Prometheus Books.

Hinman, A. R. and Hopkins, D. R. (1998), 'Lessons from Previous Eradication Programs', in Dowdle, W. R. and Hopkins, D. R. eds, *The Eradication of Infectious Diseases*, Chichester: Wiley.

Hippocrates (1973), *Hippocratic Writings* Trans. Chadwick, J. and Mann, W. N., London: Penguin.

Horstmann, D. M. (1985), 'The Poliomyelitis Story: A Scientific Hegira', *The Yale Journal of Biology and Medicine*, 58, 79–90.

———— (1991), 'The Sabin Live Poliovirus Vaccination Trials in the USSR', 1959, *Yale Journal of Biology and Medicine*, 64.

Hussain, R. S., McGarvey, S. T., Shahab, T. and Fruzzetti, L. M. (2012), 'Fatigue and Fear with Shifting Polio Eradication Strategies in India: A Study of Social Resistance to Vaccination', *PLoS ONE*, 7(9), e46274. doi:10.1371/journal.pone.0046274

IMB (2010–). Reports of the Independent Monitoring Board of the Global Polio Eradication Initiative Institute of Medicine. (1996). 'Options for Poliomyelitis Vaccination in the United States': Workshop Summary, Washington, DC.

John, T. J. (2000), 'The Final Stages of The Global Eradication of Polio', *The New England Journal of Medicine*, 343(11).

———— (2003), 'Polio Eradication in India: What is the Future?', *Indian Paediatrics*, 40(5), 455–462.

————— (2005), 'Will India need inactivated poliovirus vaccine (IPV) to complete polio eradication?', *Indian Journal of Medical Research*, 122(5), 365–367.

Kew, O., Morris-Glasgow, V., Landaverde, M., Burns, C., Shaw, J. et al (2002), 'Outbreak of Poliomyelitis in Hispaniola Associated with Circulating Type 1 Vaccine-Derived Poliovirus', *Science*, 296(5566), 356–359. doi:10.1126/science.1068284

—————, Sutter, R. W., de Gourville, E. M., Dowdle, W. R. and Pallansch, M. A. (2005), 'Vaccine-derived polioviruses and the endgame strategy for global polio eradication', *Annual Review of Microbiology*, 59, 587–635. doi:10.1146/annurev.micro.58.030603.123625

Kluger, J. (2004), 'Splendid Solution: Jonas Salk and the Conquest of Polio', New York: Berkley Publishing Group.

Kohler, K. A., Banerjee, K., Hlady, W. G., Andrus, J. K. and Sutter, R. W. (2002), 'Vaccine-associated paralytic poliomyelitis in India during 1999: Decreased risk despite massive use of oral polio vaccine', *Bulletin of the World Health Organisation*, 80(3).

—————, Banerjee, K. and Sutter, R. W. (2002), 'Further clarity on vaccine-associated paralytic polio in India', *Bulletin of the World Health Organisation*, 80(12).

Labonte, R. (2008), 'Global health in public policy: finding the right frame?', *Critical Public Health*, 18(4), 467–482. doi:10.1080/09581590802443588

Mahler, H. (1988), 'World Health 2000 and Beyond', Paper presented at the 41st World Health Assembly, Geneva.

McNeill, W. H. (1976), *Plagues and Peoples*, New York: Anchor Books.

Melnick, J. L. (1960), 'Problems Associated with the Use of Live Poliovirus Vaccine', *American Journal of Public Health*, 50(7).

Muraskin, W. (2012), *Polio Eradication and its Discontents: A Historian's Journey Through an International Public Health (Un)Civil War*, Hyderabad: Orient Blackswan.

Nathanson, N. and Kew, O. M. (2010), 'From Emergence to Eradication: The Epidemiology of Polio Deconstructed', *American Journal of Epidemiology*, 172(11).

Oshinsky, D. M. (2005), *Polio: An American Story*, New York: Oxford University Press.

Packard, R. (2007), *The Making of a Tropical Disease: A Short History of Malaria*, Baltimore, NJ: Johns Hopkins University Press.

Parks, P. J. (2004), *Jonas Salk: Polio Vaccine Pioneer*, San Diego, CA: Blackbirch Press.

Paul, J. R. (1971), *A History of Poliomyelitis*, New Haven, CT: Yale University Press.

SELECT BIBLIOGRAPHY

Pigman, H. A. (2005), *Conquering Polio: A Brief History of PolioPlus, Rotary's Role in a Global Program to Eradicate the World's Greatest Crippling Disease*, Evanston, IL: Rotary International.

Rashid, A. (2008), *Taliban: Islam, Oil and the New Great Game in Central Asia*, London: I. B. Tauris.

Rogers, N. (1992), 'Dirt and Disease Polio Before FDR Health and Medicine in American Society', Retrieved from http://eproxy.lib.hku.hk/login?url=http://www.netlibrary.com/urlapi.asp?action=summary&v=1&bookid=2066

Sabin, A. B. (1960), 'Live Orally Given Poliovirus Vaccine. Effects of Rapid Mass Immunisation on Population Under Conditions of Massive Enteric Infection With Other Viruses', *The Journal of the American Medical Association*, 173(14).

———— (1985), 'Oral Polio Vaccine: History of Its Development and Use and Current Challenge to Eliminate Poliomyelitis from the World', *The Journal of Infectious Diseases*, 151(3), 420–436.

Salk, D. and Salk, J. (1984), 'Vaccinology of Poliomyelitis', *Vaccine*, 2(1), 59–74.

Sathyamala, C., Mittal, O., Dasgupta, R. and Priya, R. (2005), 'Polio Eradication Initiative in India: Deconstructing the GPEI', *International Journal of Health Services*, 35(2), 361–383.

Shiffman, J., Beer, T. and Wu, Y. (2002), 'The Emergence of Global Disease Control Priorities', *Health Policy and Planning*, 17(3), 225–234. doi: 10.1093/heapol/17.3.225

Smallman-Raynor, M. R. and Cliff, A. D. (2006). *Poliomyelitis. A World Geography: Emergence to Eradication*, Oxford: Oxford University Press.

Smith, J. E. (2007), *FDR*, New York: Random House.

Smith, J. S. (1990), *Patenting the Sun: Polio and the Salk Vaccine*, New York: W. Morrow.

Sutter, R. W., Platt, L., Mach, O., Jafari, H. and Aylward, R. B. (2014), 'The New Polio Eradication End Game: Rationale and Supporting Evidence', *The Journal of Infectious Diseases*, 210 Suppl 1, S434–438. doi:10.1093/infdis/jiu222

Taylor, C. E., Cutts, F. and Taylor, M. E. (1997), 'Ethical Dilemmas in Current Planning for Polio Eradication', *American Journal of Public Health*, 87(6).

UNICEF, 'A Critical Leap to Polio Eradication in India', UNICEF: New Delhi.

Virchow, R. (1848), Report on the Typhus Epidemic in Upper Silesia (English Translation), *Social Medicine*, 1(1).

Ward, G. C. (2014), *A First-class Temperament: The Emergence of Franklin Roosevelt, 1905–1928*, New York: Vintage Books.

SELECT BIBLIOGRAPHY

Watts, S. (1997), *Epidemics and History: Disease, Power and Imperialism*, New Haven, CT: Yale University Press.

WHO (1988), 'Forty-First World Health Assembly Verbatim Records of Plenary Meetings Records of Committees', Paper presented at the Forty-First World Health Assembly, Geneva.

———— (1989), 'World Health Organisation Executive Board Eighty-Second Session Resolutions and Decisions Summary Records'.

———— (1989), 'Global Poliomyelitis Eradication by the Year 2000 Plan of Action', Retrieved from Geneva.

———— (1990), 'Eradication of Poliomyelitis. Report of the Third Consultation', Retrieved from Geneva.

———— (2001), 'Progress towards poliomyelitis eradication South-East Asia. Weekly Epidemiological Record', 34(76).

———— (2001), 'Thematic Evaluations in 2001 Eradication of Poliomyelitis', Report by the Director General Retrieved from Geneva.

———— (2008), 'The Third Ten Years of the World Health Organisation', Geneva: World Health Organisation.

———— (2009), 'Second Meeting of the SAGE Working Group on IPV', Retrieved from Geneva.

———— (2014), 'Information Sheet Observed Rate of Vaccine Reactions', Polio Vaccines http://www.who.int/vaccine_safety/initiative/tools/polio_vaccine_rates_information_sheet.pdf: WHO.

———— (2017), 'What is vaccine-derived polio?', retrieved from http://www.who.int/features/qa/64/en/

WHO/UNICEF (2009), 'State of the World's Vaccines and Immunisation', Third edition, Retrieved from Geneva.

Wilson, D. J., *Living With Polio: The Epidemic and its Survivors*, Chicago, IL: University of Chicago Press.

Yekutiel, P. (1981), 'Lessons from the big eradication campaigns', World Health Forum, 2(4).

ACKNOWLEDGEMENTS

This book would not have been possible without the kindness and generosity of many who have been involved in either the study of the poliovirus, or the efforts to eradicate the virus.

During my travels in Nigeria I was privileged to spend travel in Kano state with a group of UNICEF polio specialists: Lalaina Fatratra Andriamasinoro, Panchanan Achari, Mary Mendes and Deepali Sharma; Susan Mackay at UNICEF headquarters in New York opened doors to her polio team Nigeria.

In Pakistan, Azeez Memon, the long serving head of the Rotary's polio efforts in the country opened many doors for me, both in the Pakistan government as well as among fellow Rotarians. Asher Ali and Alina Vishram shared their experiences of the polio programme in Karachi, and Nowsherwan Khan was an excellent and hospitable guide to the immunisation campaigns in Rawalpindi. Elias Durry at the WHO in Pakistan and Babar bin Atta provided valuable insights into the polio programme in that country, as did Mazar Nisar Shaikh, Rana Safdar, Shahnaz Wazir Ali and Azra Pechucho. Salah Tumseh allowed me to experience the difficulties the polio programme encountered in the suburbs of Karachi.

Carol Pandak at Rotary International opened many doors in Rotary, and gave me access to meetings at the Rotary Convention in Atlanta in 2017, besides sharing her decades long experience with polio eradication. Steve Cochi, Olen Kew and Hamid Jaffri were generous with their time and knowledge, as were Sunil Bahl, Sona Bari, Deepak Kapur and Lokesh Gupta. Mathew Varghese squeezed in time to talk to

ACKNOWLEDGEMENTS

me in between surgeries at St Stephen's hospital in Delhi and help me understand the impact polio has on those it strikes.

K Sujatha Rao and Jayaprakash Muliyil provided valuable insights into some of the tensions that had crept into the polio eradication campaign in India.

I am indebted to Jacob John, one of India's polio pioneers, who unstintingly shared the knowledge of the poliovirus as well as the polio eradication campaign that he had acquired over four decades. I am grateful to Vincent Racaniello, Eckhard Wimmer, Jeronimo Cello, Olen Kew and Nicholas Grassly, giants in the study of the poliovirus and polio vaccines, for sharing their time and knowledge.

David Heymann, who, perhaps unwittingly, sparked my interest in polio eradication, was unfailingly generous with sharing his insights into the polio eradication campaign.

Turning a manuscript into a printed book is no mean task, and my thanks to Michael Dwyer at Hurst Publishers for taking a punt on this book sight unseen, and to Jon de Peyer and the rest of the team at Hurst for shepherding this through.

Last, but definitely not least, this book would not have been possible without the support of Ying Chan and then later Keith Richburg at the Journalism and Media Studies Centre at the University of Hong Kong, who gave me the time and space to work on a book that is pretty far removed from the kind of work that traditionally emerges from schools of journalism.

INDEX

Boko Haram: targeting of polio
vaccinators, 218; territory held
by, 216
Bolivia: 88
Brazil: 85, 114; polio cases in, 83;
polio immunisation campaigns
of, 88
Brennan, John: Director of CIA,
200
British Broadcasting Corporation
(BBC): 194
British Medical Journal (BMJ): 201
Brodie, Maurice: vaccination
research of, 35–6, 56
Burnet, Frank: study of poliovirus,
40
Bureau of Investigative Journalists:
198
Burundi: 54

Cabral, Dr Rodriguez: Head of
Mozambique Health Service, 119
Cambodia: Rotary vaccination
programmes in, 91
Cameroon: poliovirus in, 205
Canada: 29, 36, 71, 85
Candau, Marcelino: WHO Director
General, 101, 121
Canseco, Carlos: President of
Rotary International, 89, 93–4
Carlyle de Macedo, Guerero:
Director General of PAHO, 86,
89, 97
Center for Strategic and
International Studies: 133
Central African Republic: 129
Chad: 129, 134, 217
Chan, Margaret: WHO Director-
General, xxiv, 125, 205
China, People's Republic of: 83;
polio outbreak in, 144, 205;
Xinjiang, 205

Chisholm, Brock: WHO Director-
General, 111
chlorination: 181–2
cholera: vaccines for, 35
Christian Medical College: 179;
faculty of, 83
Chumakov, Mikhail: 67; Director
of Poliomyelitis Research
Institute, 65–6
Churchill, Winston: 49
circulating vaccine-derived polio
virus (cVDPV): concept of,
xix–xx
clinical testing: ethics of, 45
Clinton, Hillary: US Secretary of
State, 197
Cochi, Steve: 145, 177
Cold War: 28
Columbia University: 38, 149;
faculty of, 75
Committees for the Defence of the
Revolution: 69
communism: 28
Congo: 54, 134
CORE: 169
Cortez, Hernando: 18
Cote d'Ivoire: 129
Cox, Herald: 55
Crawford, Dorothy: 11
Cruz, Rodolfo Rodrigo:
Cuban National Director of
Epidemiology, 83
Cuba: 85, 114, 151; Bay of Pigs
Invasion (1961), 68; nation-
wide immunisation campaign
in (1962), 68; yellow fever
outbreaks in, 102
Cuban Missile Crisis (1962): 68
Cutter Laboratories: 64; vaccines
produced by, 37–8
Czechoslovakia: 69

Dawn: 191

INDEX